High Blood Pressure

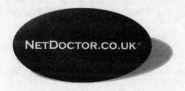

Series Editor
Dr Dan Rutherford

Hodder & Stoughton
LONDON SYDNEY AUCKLAND

**The material in this book is in no way intended to replace
professional medical care or attention by a qualified
practitioner. The materials in this book cannot and should
not be used as a basis for diagnosis or choice of treatment.**

British Library Cataloguing in Publication Data
A record for this book is available from the British Library

ISBN 0 340 78682 5

Typeset by Avon Dataset Ltd, Bidford-on-Avon, Warks

Printed and bound in Great Britain by
Bookmarque

Hodder & Stoughton
A Division of Hodder Headline Ltd
338 Euston Road
London NW1 3BH
www.madaboutbooks.com

High Blood Pressure

Contents

Foreword

High blood pressure, or in medical terms 'hypertension', is the second biggest preventable cause of death in the UK and other westernised countries. Despite this, high blood pressure rarely makes the headline news, few members of the public are aware of the importance of blood pressure, few patients with high blood pressure are aware and even some doctors are unaware. We all worry about the dangers of flying, the risks of nuclear plants or the impurities in foods but these risks are trivial when compared to the avoidable risks of high blood pressure. To put things into perspective, if the average blood pressure of the entire population could be reduced by a relatively modest amount (5 mmHg) then we could reduce the occurrence of strokes by 40 per cent and heart attacks by 20 per cent.

In the UK, high blood pressure accounts for a high proportion of consultations with family doctors and many people take blood pressure lowering tablets. Despite this, patients often admit that they know relatively little about the subject perhaps because of the low media profile. This book is intended for such patients. It is written in a style that is free from jargon but still explains things well and, where appropriate, in some detail. Ideally, every patient with high blood pressure should have a copy or at least be loaned a copy when the diagnosis is first made.

Patients often ask, 'What things can I do to help my blood pressure?' This book provides the answers. Relatively minor lifestyle changes are explained and the effect of these changes, and how to make them painlessly, are outlined.

After reading this book, patients will understand the need to 'know their numbers' i.e. they should know what their blood pressure is and know what it should be. They will understand that the risk of strokes and heart attacks increases when other risk factors are present and that reducing their overall risk is best done by a combined approach to all of these. For example, high blood cholesterol is one of the other modifiable risk factors that can be managed with diet and tablets. Another completely avoidable risk factor (and the biggest preventable cause of death in westernised countries) is the 'evil weed', cigarette smoking. Perhaps the best thing about this book is that it is interesting and easy to read. Even those without high blood pressure will find it entertaining and educational. Perhaps everyone should read it?

Professor Tom MacDonald
Hypertension Clinic and Hypertension Research Centre
Ninewells Hospital & Medical School
Dundee

Acknowledgements

A full list of people who helped in the production of this book would leave little room for the text, but special thanks are due to Professor Tom MacDonald and Dr Suzanne Wong for ensuring that the information presented here reflects current best practice in managing high blood pressure in the UK. I'm grateful also to those other medical colleagues who have reviewed the draft and made useful comments – Dr Hilary Jones, Professor Jon Rhodes, Dr Keith Barnard and Dr Bob Leckridge.

My colleagues in NetDoctor work behind the scenes and deserve more recognition – John Peel, Alex Ballantyne, Bal Singh, Jason Dunne, Matt Cook, Richard Marshall, Charlotte Ramplin, Huw Arthur, Melina Dinnis and Helen Davis, to name a few.

Judith Longman at Hodder & Stoughton is a remarkably patient editor and has been a real help at all stages from conception to delivery.

Great care has been taken to ensure that the information in this book is accurate, but if errors remain then the responsibility is mine. Please let me know if you spot any. I also welcome feedback from readers on this or any of the other books in the NetDoctor 'Help Yourself to Health' series. I can be contacted at d.rutherford@netdoctor.co.uk

Dr Dan Rutherford
Medical Director
www.netdoctor.co.uk

Chapter 1

Blood Pressure:
What It Is and Why It Matters

Introduction

If one scene typifies modern medicine it is surely the blood pressure check. The patient sits beside the doctor's desk, arm wrapped in a band attached by tubes to an odd-looking box with a graduated glass column. The doctor peers intently at the falling level of mercury behind the glass, controlling the drop with a rubber bulb in one hand, the other holding that equally symbolic medical instrument, the stethoscope, to the patient's elbow. There is silence between the two people as the doctor concentrates on the mysterious sounds only he can hear, broken gently by the hiss of air from the valve in the bulb. Then it's all over. The doctor has heard whatever was being listened for. A result has been reached, and the patient waits to hear if the conclusion is good or bad.

Blood pressure measurement is by far the most common medical test and consumes a large part of the time spent by people in contact with doctors and nurses, and vice versa. The level of a person's blood pressure can have profound health implications and millions of people worldwide take medical treatment for raised pressure. The global medical industry, both academic and commercial, involved with the research and treatment of this single aspect of human biology engages hundreds of thousands of people, and billions of pounds of expenditure.

At its simplest level, blood pressure is an easy enough concept to understand. The heart is a pump designed to force blood through the miles of piping of our blood vessels, and pumps work by generating pressure. Too much pressure puts a strain on the piping and on the pump itself, which might cause a pipe to burst or the pump to fail under the strain – in the worst case stopping altogether. The science of blood pressure control is now a vast body of complex medical literature, but this simple analogy fits well with many of the observed consequences of high blood pressure.

To understand more fully what blood pressure is all about, we need to take each part of the process in turn and look at it in more detail. The aim of this book is to help you understand blood pressure and its control, what the problems of abnormal blood pressure are and why we think they occur, and the reasoning behind blood pressure treatment. If you have high blood pressure, or know someone who does, this book should help you feel better informed about the condition, and what can be done to keep healthy while living with it.

One of the problems with medical subjects is that they are often accompanied by jargon, and this will be explained as it crops up. Now is a good time to start. 'Hypertension' is one word that means 'high blood pressure' and someone with hypertension is referred to by doctors as 'hypertensive'. Drugs for high blood pressure are often called 'anti-hypertensives'. Low blood pressure's shorthand term is 'hypotension', and as anti-hypertensive drugs always lower blood pressure one way or another they are said to have a 'hypotensive effect' on blood pressure. Getting these terms in our heads now will be helpful later.

Measuring blood pressure

We'll look in detail at this in chapter 4, but a brief summary at this stage will let us understand why high blood pressure is so important. All references to blood pressure levels quote the unit of measurement as 'millimetres of mercury', abbreviated to 'mmHg'. To understand the principle of pressure measurement take a look at figure 1.

At the top of the diagram, in figure 1 (A), there is a table on top of which rests a tank of water on the left. From the bottom of the tank exits a flexible tube. There is also an empty beaker resting on the tube and for the purpose of our imaginary experiment we'll let this be made of a weightless material. The tube is made of a super-flexible material, so the only thing keeping it open is the pressure of the water within it. Water comes out of the end of the tube at a rate depending on the height of the water in the tank because the more water is in the tank, the greater is the force of gravity at the point where the tube is attached, and the greater is the force, or pressure, of water in the tube. It's important to realise that the width of the tank of water is not important – only the depth. To take an example, if you were to dive to 10 metres down in a swimming pool, the pressure of water around you would be just the same as if you were at 10 metres in a lake – only the depth matters, not the size of the pool.

In figure 1 (B) water has been added to the beaker, the weight of which is pressing down on the tube, trying to close it. So long as the height of water in the tank (keeping the tube open) is greater than that in the beaker (trying to close the tube), then the tube pressure will be high enough to remain open and water will flow. When the levels of water in tank and beaker are equal the opening (tank) and closing (beaker) pressures are exactly balanced. If one more drop of water is added to the beaker it will make the closing pressure greater than the tube pressure, so the tube will be flattened by the beaker and the flow of water will stop.

In figure 1 (C) the water in the beaker has been replaced with mercury – over 13 times more dense than water and in fact the densest of all liquids. Now the closing pressure on the tube can be achieved

Figure 1: Principle of blood pressure measurement

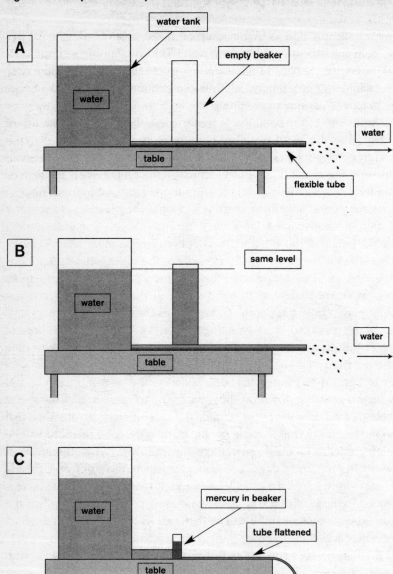

with a small beaker of mercury – less than one thirteenth of the height of the water.

This is pretty much exactly how a blood pressure measuring device, or 'sphygmomanometer' (pronounced 'sfig-mo-manometer') to give it its proper title, works. In the experiment, the pump was the large tank and the pressure forcing water out of the bottom pipe was the effect of gravity. In a human being the pump is the heart, which generates pressure with every beat. The flexible tube is, in real life, a main artery in the arm – the 'brachial' artery – which is conveniently situated in the middle of the bend of the elbow. Placing a stethoscope here lets the doctor listen to the flow of blood through the arm. Finally, the beaker of mercury is replaced by the column in the sphygmomanometer, the

Figure 2: Set up for measuring blood pressure

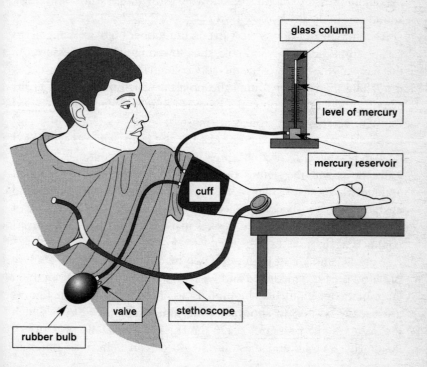

pressure of which is transmitted to the patient's arm by the cuff wrapped around it – see figure 2.

To take a blood pressure reading the doctor pumps up the pressure within a flat rubber bladder (called the 'cuff') wrapped around the patient's upper arm using a rubber bulb connected to the bladder by a tube and valve arrangement. Another tube leads from the bladder to a reservoir of mercury at the bottom of a vertical glass column, which is marked out in millimetre divisions. Whatever pressure is present in the cuff is therefore shown on the mercury column. The mercury is held within a sealed system – only air travels in the rubber tubing and the cuff. When the pressure in the cuff is less than the pressure of blood being forced through the artery by the beating of the heart the doctor can clearly hear the pulse with a stethoscope over the front of the elbow. When the pressure is pumped up above the heart's maximum pressure, blood stops flowing through the arm, so no pulse sound can be heard at the elbow.

Then the doctor opens the valve in the rubber bulb, allowing air to escape from the tubing and cuff, thus lowering the cuff pressure. As this happens the height of the mercury column falls. The doctor watches the falling mercury level until the point at which the pulse is heard again is noted. At this point the heart is just managing to pump blood through, so the heart's pressure must be equal to that of the cuff pressure. This is the maximum pressure the heart achieves with each beat and is called the 'systolic' pressure. The doctor continues to listen to the pulse with the stethoscope while the pressure is allowed to fall and records another reading – the 'diastolic' pressure – when the sound character alters to become quieter. This is in effect the low point of pressure in the body's blood vessels that occurs just before the heart contracts again in its next beat.

'Systolic' and 'diastolic' are the two main words in the vocabulary of blood pressure medicine and we'll go into more detail about them later. In the meantime it is helpful just to know the terms. The figures are usually written in shorthand, like this example: 120/90, which means a systolic pressure of 120 mmHg and a diastolic pressure of 90 mmHg. Systolic and diastolic pressures can behave in different ways, which is why both readings are always taken and are important to know.

By using such a dense liquid as mercury the sphygmomanometer can be made much more compact than is possible with other liquids – water could be used but to cope with the range of blood pressure in human beings the glass column would need to be at least 3 metres high! One can imagine the antics necessary of the doctor or nurse reading a three metre high tube while trying to listen for the pulse (not to mention the need for consulting rooms with high ceilings) and readily accept why mercury has always been the favourite choice for this instrument. It requires only gravity to work, and gravity is virtually equal all over the world, so the mercury-based instrument has allowed a consistent global standard to be applied to blood pressure measurement. However, mercury is also a potentially dangerous material – it can be absorbed through the skin and readily evaporates to produce toxic mercury vapour, so spillages have to be taken seriously. Mercury sphygmomanometers are robust but they can be broken or leak, so they are being phased out and replaced with electronic devices. The unit of blood pressure measurement is nonetheless likely to remain 'mmHg' for a very long time to come.

Blood pressure and the individual

Blood pressure is not constant in individuals over the course of their lives. Leaving aside those who develop abnormalities of blood pressure, even those whose pressure is deemed 'normal' will show a tendency for their pressure to rise with age. This is illustrated in figure 3. Healthy adults in their early twenties show a systolic pressure in the range 115–125 mmHg but in their late sixties show readings around 140–145 mmHg. There is a similar upwards drift in diastolic pressure from about 70 mmHg to 85 mmHg in the same age groups. This pattern of blood pressure rising with age is seen only in 'developed' countries, and probably reflects our high intake of salt and trend to becoming overweight. At all ages until about 60 onwards men tend to have higher pressures than women. Elderly women however have

Figure 3: Increase of blood pressure with age

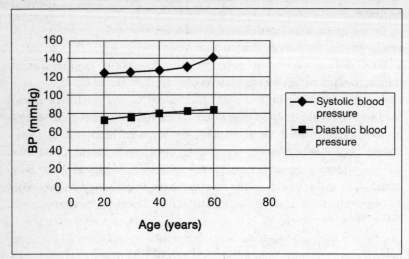

slightly higher pressures than men, and are more likely to have hypertension too.

Blood pressure and populations

I've mentioned that Western-style diets seem to increase blood pressure with time, but there are other observed differences between population groups. Black people tend to show higher blood pressures than whites and the health problems associated with hypertension are more pronounced in the black population. Hypertension is common in Japan but results more often in stroke than in heart disease (see the next section on health risks) because the traditional Japanese diet is low in fat and high in salt. Japanese who move to the USA and adopt American eating habits eat more fat and less salt, and then start to show more heart disease but fewer strokes. People from the Indian subcontinent are particularly prone to developing heart disease.

In all these populations there is a complex mixture of different factors – cultural and geographical differences in diets, attitudes to exercise, access to health care and other factors – many of which we have yet to discover and understand, which determine someone's blood pressure and the health risks associated with it.

Definition of hypertension

As soon as one tries to define what is 'normal' and 'abnormal' blood pressure one hits a difficulty, common to many biological measurements, which is that there is no clear distinction between the two groups. Take height as an appropriate example of the same problem. Measurements of the heights of several thousand adults selected at random will show a pattern similar to that in figure 4. Most people will

Figure 4: Distribution of height in a population

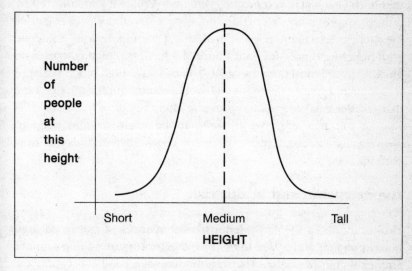

be at or near the middle of the range, whereas there will be progressively fewer people who are very short or very tall. The majority of people will be perfectly 'normal' as far as their height is concerned

– only a small proportion will be very tall or very short for a medical reason such as a hormone problem – and there is certainly no clear line between 'normal' and 'abnormal' height.

A graph of the blood pressures of the same group of people would look very similar, with the minority of people showing readings at the high or low end of the range and most people somewhere in the middle. To determine whether blood pressure is 'too high' we need information that tells us what are the consequences for health for any given level of blood pressure. In other words, a good definition of hypertension would be the level of blood pressure at which our health starts to be affected for the worse.

Symptoms of high blood pressure

One of the most important things to remember about hypertension is that in the early stages *it has no symptoms*. Unlike a joint affected by arthritis, there is no pain. High blood pressure almost never causes headaches, despite the popular myth that it commonly does. Someone with high blood pressure looks normal – having a 'high colour' is no guide to your blood pressure at all. You can have high blood pressure for years and feel perfectly fit and well. Finding out for the first time that someone has high blood pressure after they have had a stroke is finding out too late. We all need to be aware of the need to periodically have our blood pressure checked, regardless of how well we feel.

Hypertension and health risk

Stroke is one of the most serious consequences of untreated high blood pressure and is due to the blockage or rupture of one or more arteries within the brain. The resulting damage can be very serious, with loss of speech and paralysis being common, or it can be fatal – stroke is one of the most common causes of death in the UK. The relationship between blood pressure and the risk of having a stroke is shown in figure 5.

Figure 5: Risk of stroke in hypertension

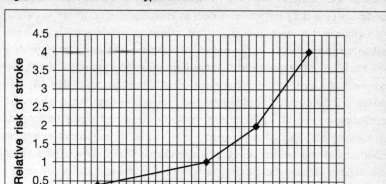

Blood pressure is marked along the horizontal axis of the graph in figure 5 and the vertical axis shows the risk of stroke. In this study the average diastolic blood pressure reading for the whole group was 91 mmHg – this point has been marked on the graph. The curved line on the graph maps this blood pressure figure against the number 1.0 on the vertical axis – this represents the average risk of stroke for the group. The effect on stroke risk of other levels of blood pressure is quite dramatic. Someone with a blood pressure of 98 mmHg – just a 7 mmHg increase, has about double the risk (2.0 on the vertical scale). A pressure of 105 mmHg has four times the risk (4.0 on vertical scale). However, a diastolic pressure of 76 mmHg has less than half the stroke risk of 91 mmHg.

A graph showing the risk of developing angina and heart attacks from high blood pressure looks very similar although not quite as steep as that for stroke. Many such studies over the past fifty years have conclusively proved that high blood pressure is significantly associated with major health risks. As will be shown later, the chances of these health problems occurring is increased by the presence of other factors such as smoking, raised blood cholesterol, diabetes and obesity, along with high blood pressure.

Hopefully it is now clear that 'hypertension' is something we have had to work to define – it is not as straightforward or as definite as a broken bone. The definition of hypertension has changed over the past twenty–thirty years, as we have better understood the adverse effects, particularly of mildly elevated blood pressure, on health. The late Professor Geoffrey Rose, who was Professor of Epidemiology at the London School of Hygiene and Tropical Medicine, defined hypertension as 'that level of blood pressure above which investigation and treatment do more good than harm' and it remains a valid definition.

We now know that people with systolic blood pressure consistently above 160 mmHg need treatment and those with diastolic pressure above 100 mmHg (and probably above 90 mmHg) do too. Both systolic and diastolic pressure are important – either one being elevated to these levels merits treatment even if the other is normal. The aim of treatment is to achieve systolic pressure below 140 mmHg and diastolic pressure below 85 mmHg on a permanent basis.

Other risks of hypertension

Although strokes and heart attacks are the most serious events that we know can be caused by hypertension, there are many others of importance. 'Heart failure' literally means that the heart begins to fail as a pump, and hypertension is the main known cause. In a large research study carried out in the USA (known as the 'Framingham Study' – see appendix A for references) people with blood pressures over 160/95 mmHg were three to four times more likely to develop heart failure than those whose pressures were less than 140/90 mmHg. Heart failure causes breathlessness on walking about, swelling of the feet and ankles and congestion of the lungs from the build up of too much fluid within the body – like a wet sponge.

Arteries are the tubes that take blood from the heart to all parts of the body. When we are young and healthy they are flexible and wide, but as we get older they tend to develop thicker walls and to become less flexible. As a result blood finds it harder to get through them. The common term for this is 'hardening of the arteries' (the proper medical term is 'atherosclerosis'). When atherosclerosis affects the arteries of the legs then a person will have difficulty walking long distances without having to stop because of muscle aches. The aches are due to the muscles running out of nutrients such as oxygen, as the blood supply can't keep up with their needs. After a few minutes rest the person can usually walk on the same distance before needing the next rest. Hypertension makes this twice as likely to develop in a man and nearly four times more likely in a woman compared with individuals with normal blood pressure.

Many people who develop severe atherosclerosis of the main artery of the body – the aorta – also have hypertension. Although atherosclerosis hardens arteries it also weakens them – the flexible blood vessels of youth are stronger than the stiff arteries of old age, which in the case of the aorta can cause it to balloon out into an 'aneurysm' – a bulging segment that can be at risk of rupture, with potentially fatal consequences.

Hypertension also damages the small arteries throughout the body, narrowing them and reducing the blood flow to the tissues they serve. The consequences vary with the organ involved. In the brain multiple 'mini-strokes' can lead to dementia, in the kidneys severe hypertension is a major cause of kidney failure and in the back part of the eye (the retina or light-sensitive part) the small arteries that cross the surface of the retina to supply it with blood can rupture, leak or become blocked. Impairment of sight due to high blood pressure alone is, fortunately, fairly uncommon except when there has been blockage (thrombosis) of one of the small arteries or veins of the retina.

Although hypertension can cause many health problems, it does so almost entirely through the damage it causes to the body's arteries and heart – the 'cardiovascular system'. Hypertension does not influence the likelihood of getting cancer, asthma, arthritis, mental illness or other common medical conditions.

MULTIPLE RISKS

It has become clear to medical researchers for several decades that it is much more useful to look at hypertension as one of several factors that can affect an individual's risk of developing cardiovascular disease rather than considering it on its own. This of course is also common sense – a fit non-smoker who is at his ideal weight and takes regular exercise is not the same as someone who smokes, is obese and takes

Figure 6: Interaction of the main risk factors for heart disease

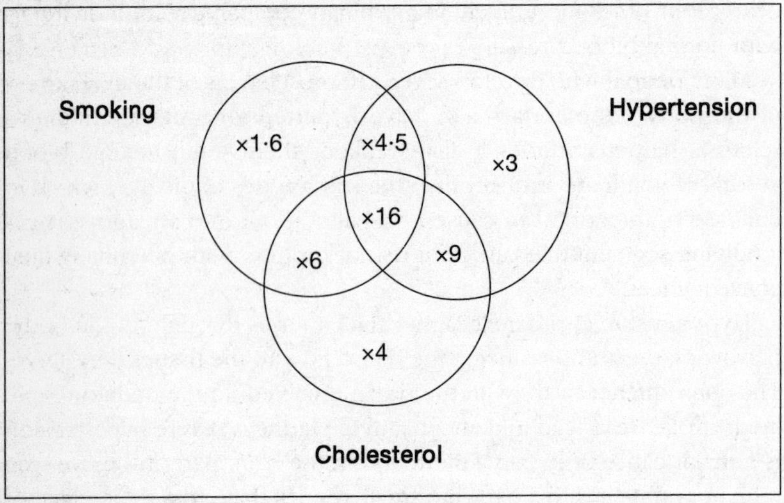

no exercise even if they both have raised blood pressures to the same degree. When we look at the combined effects of multiple risk factors we can see clearly how important it is to take the whole person into consideration, rather than a single measurement. This should be the aim of all good medical practice but too often it is neglected under the time pressures typical within the health service. Look at figure 6, which illustrates the interplay of three main risk factors that we can modify (as opposed to those that we cannot modify, such as our sex or race).

In the figure there are three circles – one each for hypertension, smoking and raised cholesterol – and you will see that they all overlap. The numbers within each main area represent the increase in risk of developing coronary heart disease that would be experienced by a middle-aged non-smoker with normal blood pressure and blood cholesterol were he to have any of these three risk factors:

- Systolic blood pressure of 195 mmHg
- Blood cholesterol raised to 8.25 mmol/l or more
- Smoking to any extent.

For example, if this person took up smoking he would increase his chance of getting coronary heart disease by 1.6 times. If his cholesterol went up to 8.25 mmol/l his risk would increase by 4 times. If he had both raised cholesterol and smoked the risk would be 6 times greater – the overlap between the two areas. In the middle is someone with all three risk factors, whose risk is 16 times greater than the low-risk individual. This diagram makes it clear not only that multiple risk factors greatly increase the likelihood of coronary heart disease, but also that removing a modifiable risk factor is very beneficial.

If our 'man in the middle' stopped smoking and did nothing else his risk would in theory improve from x16 to x9 – a very considerable drop. Even better than stopping smoking is never starting. In the Medical Research Council trial of the treatment of mild hypertension the importance of having never smoked outweighed any benefit from treatment to lower blood pressure.

Modifiable and non-modifiable risk factors are looked at in more detail in chapters 3 and 7, along with tips on how you can assess your own risk and in chapter 8 there is information on how to improve modifiable risk factors.

The benefits of treating hypertension

The previous pages may have left you with a sense of doom and gloom, particularly if you suffer from hypertension, with their information about the problems that can result – but that was not the intention.

Hypertension is treatable and the benefits of doing so are now well established. The figures are most dramatic for the most severe form of hypertension – so called 'malignant hypertension' (which has nothing to do with cancer but uses the word malignant to mean a condition which is life-threatening without treatment).

Malignant hypertension is uncommon and refers to a type of hypertension that rapidly gets worse, with diastolic blood pressures over 120 mmHg (i.e. levels that would normally only apply to systolic pressure) accompanied by kidney and brain damage and probably heart failure too. Prior to the arrival of effective anti-hypertensive drugs malignant hypertension was usually fatal within months, but now 85 per cent of such patients are curable and lead healthy lives. The benefits of treating milder hypertension are perhaps less dramatic but still impressive. Reducing diastolic blood pressure by about 5 or 6 mmHg over a period of five years would in theory reduce the risk of stroke by 40 per cent and the risk of heart attack by about 20 per cent. Achieving such modest reduction in blood pressure is definitely possible, and if it were done across the general population of hypertensive people there would be enormous benefits both to the individuals and to society.

STROKE

Hypertension is not the only cause of strokes and heart attacks, so treating high blood pressure cannot eliminate all occurrences of either condition. Thirty-five to forty per cent of strokes are however thought to be directly due to hypertension, so the potential reduction of 40 per cent of strokes with treatment for high blood pressure means that virtually all strokes due to hypertension are preventable. This holds good for patients up to the age of about 80 years, so previous ideas that older people with high blood pressure were best left alone are wrong. Not every 79 year old with raised blood pressure will necessarily be able to take or benefit from anti-hypertensive treatment – we still need the skill of the doctor to make a good judgement in an individual's case – but age alone is no reason to ignore the blood pressure reading.

A major study is currently under way involving several research centres across Europe to determine the effectiveness of treating hypertension in those over 80 (the Hypertension in the Very Elderly, or HYVET study) but the information gleaned from those older people who were involved with other research studies suggests that they too had their stroke risk reduced by treatment. There is some evidence that dementia developing from mini-strokes caused by hypertension can be slowed down by blood pressure control.

HEART DISEASE

The results of hypertension treatment on the occurrence of heart disease have shown slightly smaller benefits (about 16 per cent reduction of heart attacks) than theoretically predicted (20–25 per cent), probably because of more complex biological reasons behind the development of coronary artery disease compared to stroke that we don't yet fully understand. Effective anti-hypertensive treatment can reverse the development of heart failure or of a pulse abnormality called atrial fibrillation when these have been brought on by hypertension.

Key Points

- Hypertension is the medical term for high blood pressure.
- 'Systolic' is the maximum pressure of blood in each heartbeat.
- 'Diastolic' is the minimum pressure of blood in each heartbeat.
- Blood pressure is measured in millimetres of mercury, written as mmHg.
- There is no clear dividing line between normal and abnormal blood pressure. High blood pressure is defined as the level at which it causes other medical problems to occur.
- Hypertension is common in the developed world and less common in those parts of the world where less salt is consumed in the diet.
- The main risks of high blood pressure are an increased likelihood of stroke and heart attack
- The presence of other risk factors, such as smoking or raised cholesterol, increases the risks of hypertension.

Chapter 2

How the Body Controls Blood Pressure

The ways in which the body controls blood pressure may not yet be fully understood but we do now have a good working idea of the various parts of the jigsaw. It is a complex and elegant system involving the heart, brain, nervous system, hormone-producing glands, kidneys, lungs and blood vessels, to name the most important parts! Knowing a bit about the structure of the blood vessel system of the body and the details of blood pressure biology is very helpful in trying to understand why high (and low) blood pressure occurs and how lifestyle changes and anti-hypertensive treatment can be used keep blood pressure normal.

The heart and blood vessel system

The heart beats 100,000 times a day on average, and each time sends a charge of blood into the myriad of tubes that make up our arteries.

The largest artery in the body, the aorta, is 3 to 4 cm in diameter where it originates at the heart, and all other arteries in the body start as a branch of the aorta, then progressively divide like the limbs of a tree until every part of the body has been reached.

The smallest arteries are the arterioles – fractions of a millimetre across, they in turn divide to become the capillaries, the smallest blood vessels of all. Capillaries are about 7.5 microns (thousandths of a millimetre) in diameter – just wide enough to let through the red cells of the blood. Red cells carry oxygen from the lungs and, having done the job of delivering the oxygen where it is needed, they take up carbon dioxide – the waste product released when cells use glucose for fuel. Then the capillaries join up again in progressively larger vessels to form veins that deliver blood back to the heart, completing the circuit.

An adult human has about 60,000 miles of capillaries, with a total surface area of 1,000 m² – greater than three tennis courts. This is such a large network that we don't have enough blood to completely fill every part of it all the time. The function of arterioles, under the command of hormones and the nervous system, is to control the flow of blood to the capillary system. This is possible because arterioles are not simply small pipes passively conducting blood but are active structures with specialised muscle in their walls. Contraction and relaxation of these muscles narrows or opens the arteriole thus controlling the flow of blood through it.

It is a fact of physics, familiar to anyone who has tried to empty a bicycle pump while holding their thumb over the exit hole, that when a fluid or gas is forced through an opening it takes more effort to go through a narrow hole than a wide one. This is because the resistance to flow through a tube increases as the tube narrows. Applying this principle to the circulatory system the amount of force, and hence blood pressure, required of the heart to get blood round the body depends very much on the width of the millions of arterioles throughout the body. When resistance is increased, blood pressure goes up, and when it is lowered, blood pressure drops. We will shortly look at the mechanisms for the control of arteriole size, but this is one of the main controlling factors in blood pressure value. In medical circles it is called 'peripheral resistance'.

In life the arterioles throughout the body do not act the same way simultaneously – if they did and the command went out for them all to open wide our blood pressure would fall so much that we would immediately faint. The body is of course cleverer than that. The arteriole system is actively managed so that blood is diverted to tissues where it is needed most and reduced in other regions according to circumstance. A good example is exercise, where the blood flow within muscles may be 10 times greater than it is at rest and the flow to some internal organs such as the digestive system will simultaneously decrease in order to make blood available. Of course during exercise the heart rate also increases, which serves to increase the supply of blood to all tissues.

An increase in heart rate on its own, provided all of the arterioles remain constant in size, will increase blood pressure – more blood per second is trying to get through tubes of the same diameter and this can only happen if the force driving the blood through increases. This is the second controlling factor in blood pressure – the 'cardiac output'. The balance between cardiac output and peripheral resistance determines the actual blood pressure.

The biology of blood pressure control

There are numerous known parts in the biological systems we have to control our blood pressure. I'll cover these individually now and at the end of this chapter will try to show how they interact with each other.

1 THE NERVOUS SYSTEM

We are reasonably familiar with the concept of a nerve running to a muscle, and conducting a signal arising in the brain that tells the muscle to contract. Thus we can carry out a voluntary action like running for a bus or combing our hair. That is the function of the 'somatic' nervous system, whose nerves also include those of sensation, hearing and sight.

The 'autonomic' nervous system is the other part of the body's nerve network but is much more the unsung hero. Unlike the somatic nervous system, the autonomic system is generally not under our voluntary command. It is responsible for controlling our breathing, temperature, digestion, bladder, bowels, blood pressure and all the other regulatory functions that keep our internal environment stable.

Although nerves are a bit like electrical cables in the way they conduct messages they in fact use a combination of electrical impulses and chemical 'messengers' to deliver their signal. At the end of all nerves, where they reach the tissue with which they are connected, the nerve ending splays out to form a highly specialised connection zone – the end plate – which is very close to, but does not touch, the tissue cell. This is illustrated in figure 7, and uses a voluntary muscle as an example.

Figure 7: Nerve–muscle connection

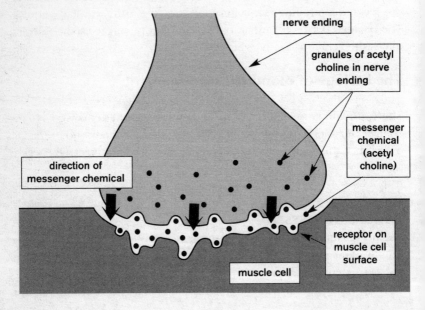

Remember that the scale of this is extremely small – of the order of a few microns across. Within the end plate of the nerve there are 'packets' of the signalling chemical – in the case of voluntary muscle this is 'acetyl choline' – held in readiness. Upon the arrival of the signal at the nerve ending the nerve releases tiny amounts of acetyl choline from these granules, which cross the gap to connect with receptors on the muscle side of the junction. These receptors are specifically shaped proteins that recognise acetyl choline just as a lock recognises the correct key. When that happens the signal to the muscle fibre is triggered, and it contracts.

Both the somatic and the autonomic nervous systems use this method of nerve signalling, but the somatic system uses only acetyl choline as its messenger chemical – the autonomic system also uses two other chemicals – noradrenaline and nitric oxide. With that background under our belt, we can move on.

There are two parts to the autonomic nervous system – the 'parasympathetic' and 'sympathetic'. The **parasympathetic** system largely comprises the vagus nerve and all its connections. This nerve arises at the base of the brain and travels throughout the chest and abdomen, sending branches to the lungs, gut, gall bladder, urinary bladder and the heart. The connections to the heart use acetyl choline as the signalling chemical and when the vagus nerve is stimulated, the heart rate slows down.

This is the basis of fainting when someone is subjected to severe shock or pain. Such strong stimuli cause a marked increase in activity of the vagus nerve; slowing the heart and reducing the blood pressure. If the heart slows too much the blood pressure falls so low that insufficient blood reaches the brain, causing loss of consciousness. Then the body's protective mechanism, which is simple but effective, makes us fall to the floor whereupon blood quickly returns to the brain and recovery occurs.

The **sympathetic** system is a chain of linked nerves that run the length of the spine on either side. Connected at multiple levels with the spinal cord, further nerve branches go to the pupils of the eye, salivary glands, lungs, heart, gut, bladder, liver and important hormone-producing glands which lie on the top of each kidney, called the adrenal glands. Most importantly for our understanding of blood pressure control, the sympathetic nervous system extends fibres throughout the walls of the whole system of arteries of the body and when these nerves are active they cause the muscle within the arterial walls to contract and therefore cause them to become narrower. The predominant chemical messenger used by the sympathetic nervous system is noradrenaline.

In many ways the sympathetic and parasympathetic systems act in opposite ways to each other. Action of the sympathetic system on the heart stimulates it to speed up and sympathetic action on arterioles causes them to narrow, both of which cause a rise in blood pressure. The parasympathetic nervous system slows the heart, which lowers the blood pressure – it has very little effect upon arteriole size.

There are two more ways in which the autonomic system influences blood pressure. The adrenal glands, of which we have two – one above each kidney – are part of the sympathetic nervous system. They have many actions but the one with which we are concerned here is the production of the hormone adrenaline (which is chemically similar to noradrenaline). The adrenal glands discharge their hormone output straight into the blood stream, and when adrenaline reaches the heart it causes it to speed up. So stimulation of the sympathetic nervous system can speed up the heart directly – by the nerve fibres that go straight to it – and indirectly through the action of adrenaline in the bloodstream.

Already it is clear that blood pressure control is a complicated affair, but there is more to come. It is worth persevering though, as it will begin to make sense shortly!

2 THE RENIN-ANGIOTENSIN SYSTEM

Renin is a hormone that circulates in the blood and is manufactured by special cells within the kidneys that are sensitive to blood pressure. If blood pressure falls these cells increase their production of renin. Also circulating in the blood is a compound called angiotensinogen, which by itself has no effect on blood pressure. In the presence of renin however angiotensinogen is converted to angiotensin I. Angiotensin I also has no effect on blood pressure but is converted within the lungs by an enzyme present there, called angiotensin converting enzyme (ACE), into angiotensin II. Angiotensin II has a powerful narrowing effect on arterioles – in fact it is one of the most potent compounds yet discovered that can do this. The 'renin-angiotensin system' is probably the most important mechanism the body uses to control blood pressure. It would be wonderfully simple if we found that disturbance of the renin-angiotensin system was the cause of hypertension, but in fact this does not appear to be the case. As we will see shortly, the majority of people with hypertension do not have an identifiable cause for it. In addition to the general effect of the renin-angiotensin system through-out the body there is evidence to suggest that local renin systems exist within individual organs such as the heart to control local blood flow.

3 THE LINING OF ARTERIES

The highly specialised cells lining the arteries are known as the 'endothelium'. This thin layer is very important, because these cells manufacture molecules which are known to constrict arteries, such as endothelin (also called ET-1) and to open arteries, such as nitric oxide. Although we know that these mechanisms exist, and that they are very important in controlling blood flow to regions of the capillary system, it's not yet known how they matter when someone develops high blood pressure.

4 CALCIUM AND MUSCLE CELLS

The more we reveal of how living cells work the more we have to marvel at. Each individual cell of the body needs to maintain its own internal chemical environment so that the processes of life such as energy use, cell repair and division and the specific functions of tissue cells can be carried out. This is engineering at the molecular level, and the cell membrane is a good example. The membrane of a cell is its surrounding wall. Far from being an inert container to keep the cell contents tidy the cell membrane is intensely active and carries out numerous chemical processes.

Within cells the concentration of electrically charged atoms (ions) is of great importance to their function. Taking muscle cells as an example, the concentration of calcium ions within the muscle cell is kept lower than the fluid outside the cell by 'pumps' within the cell membrane. When a muscle cell is triggered to contract the process involves the opening of calcium channels within the membrane – atomic gates we could say – that allow calcium to flood into the cell, thus stimulating it to contract. Once the contraction phase is over the cell is restored to the relaxed state by the calcium pumps, which transport the excess calcium within the cell back to the outside. This is what happens to the muscle cells lining arteries, so making calcium very important to blood pressure. By blocking the calcium channels using specially designed drugs the arterioles can be stopped from contracting, which lowers blood pressure.

5 HEART HORMONES

The two main pumping chambers of the heart are the 'ventricles'. Composed entirely of muscle they are separated from each other by the dividing wall within the heart that separates it into right and left halves. They look a bit like two half-dome shapes placed flat sides together. The ventricles relax when filling with blood and then contract powerfully in unison with each pulse, ejecting blood into the artery connected to each. The right ventricle takes blood returning from the body and pumps it through both lungs, where it picks up fresh oxygen. The left ventricle accepts this refreshed blood from the lungs and pumps it back to the body through the aorta – the largest artery in the body. The muscle of the left ventricle is considerably thicker and stronger than that of the right ventricle as it is a lot more work to push blood round the body than only through the lungs. Each ventricle has a small antechamber, called the (right or left) atrium, which acts as a reservoir for incoming blood. Each atrium is also made of muscle and is separate from its neighbour. The heart's internal pacemaker triggers both atria to contract together at the end of the filling phase of the ventricles. This sends an extra surge of blood into the ventricles, filling them fully prior to the next beat. It is the biological equivalent of a supercharger in a car engine, which blows air and petrol into each cylinder prior to ignition.

Within the walls of each atrium there are cells sensitive to being stretched and which manufacture and release a hormone called atrial natriuretic peptide (ANP) into the bloodstream. ANP is a diuretic i.e. a substance that stimulates the kidneys to produce more urine. ANP helps control the volume of blood in our circulation – if too much blood is circulating then the stretch-sensitive cells will become more stretched, release more ANP and the kidneys will get rid of more fluid from the circulation, as urine. Blood volume will then fall. ANP also relaxes the muscle of arterioles and reduces the body's manufacture of renin and another important hormone made by the adrenal glands called aldosterone. All of these actions lower blood pressure. The ventricles too produce a similar hormone – confusingly called brain natriuretic peptide (BNP) as it was first discovered in brain tissue. The fact that the heart itself manufactures hormones and is more than a sophisticated pump is another of the remarkable facts discovered by research into blood pressure control.

6 ALDOSTERONE AND OTHER HORMONES

Aldosterone is a hormone produced by the adrenal glands in response to stimulation from the autonomic nervous system and also by the action of angiotensin II circulating in the blood. It stimulates the kidneys to reclaim sodium that would otherwise be discharged in the urine. Sodium is the common salt in our diet and is critical in blood pressure control. In effect sodium and water go hand in hand in the body. Reclaiming sodium means also reclaiming water, so aldosterone acts to increase blood volume and pressure.

One other hormone deserves a mention, this time produced by the pituitary gland of the brain. This is antidiuretic hormone (ADH). As its name implies ADH acts on the kidneys to reduce their output of urine so, like aldosterone, it can potentially raise blood pressure too. ADH output can also be stimulated by angiotensin II.

7 SALT AND BLOOD PRESSURE

A large amount of scientific evidence shows clearly that there is a direct relationship between high intake of salt in the diet and high blood pressure. Cutting down the amount of dietary salt is an effective way of lowering blood pressure without drugs. Sodium is essential for life and the amount within the body is dependent not only on how much we eat of it, but also on the activity of a sodium-saving process carried out by the kidneys. The kidneys act continuously to filter our blood, removing soluble waste products and passing them into urine for discharge from the body. In this process of filtering sodium also passes into the urine, but a biochemical 'sodium pump' within the kidney reclaims this sodium and returns it to the bloodstream. The activity of this pump therefore controls the loss of sodium and ultimately the amount of sodium in the body. This is how aldosterone works – it is the hormone controlling the action of the sodium pump. If there is too much aldosterone then the kidney reclaims too much sodium. Bearing in mind that with sodium comes water, then hypertension can occur.

How it works together

In real life the many systems involved in blood pressure control work smoothly together, adapting the blood pressure to the body's needs. When we are asleep in bed, lying flat, our blood pressure and pulse rate are at their lowest. They rise when we rise, and when we need to rush they speed up appropriately. It's helpful to think of the body needing to adapt blood pressure at two rates – sometimes very quickly, perhaps over a few seconds, to allow a burst of speed for example, or more slowly – over weeks if necessary – when bringing the pressure back into line following an event such as blood loss (figure 8).

Figure 8: Diagram of systems involved in blood pressure control

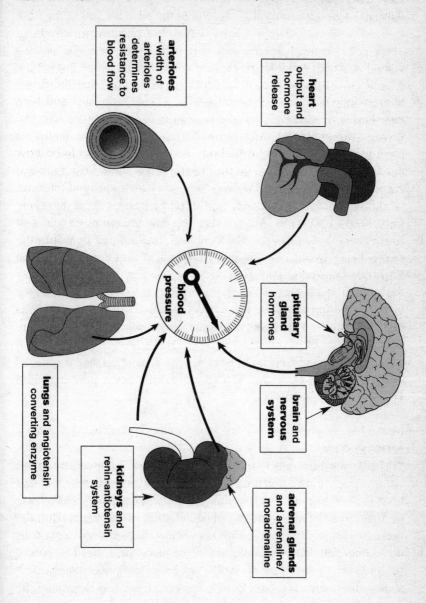

FAST SYSTEM

Specially adapted nerve cells exist within the main arteries of the neck (carotid arteries) and in the aorta, which are sensitive to stretching. These cells – called baroreceptors – are part of the autonomic nervous system and with every heartbeat they send signals, depending on the degree to which they have been stretched, to the control centre at the base of the brain. When blood pressure goes up, they are more stretched with each beat, so they send more signals to the brain. The reverse is true if the blood pressure falls. In effect they are biological pressure gauges. The brain in turn sends signals to the rest of the nerve system that dictate the state of the pulse (cardiac output) and arteriole width (peripheral resistance).

Should we stand up quickly our blood pressure will fall as gravity pulls blood down towards our feet but this lowers the amount of stretch on the baroreceptors, which sets off a train of signals in the sympathetic part of the autonomic nervous system commanding the heart rate to increase and arterioles to contract. Within a few seconds our blood pressure has been adjusted upwards to cope with standing.

The opposite happens when we lie down – sympathetic nerve activity is lowered, and parasympathetic activity is increased, slowing our pulse.

Should we need an extra burst of activity then adrenaline is released from the adrenal gland and carried around the body, boosting pulse rate and blood pressure.

SLOW SYSTEM

This involves the kidneys, with their production of renin and its effects on angiotensin, the stretch receptors in the heart producing ANP and BNP, the production of aldosterone by the adrenal glands and release of antidiuretic hormone by the pituitary gland of the brain. All these processes involve the synthesis of hormones and their knock-on effects on sodium and water balance, and hence blood pressure. This part of the pressure control process works over a much longer time scale – some adjustments take weeks to complete. They also determine the overall blood pressure more significantly than the short-term effects of the baroreceptors. Drugs to control blood pressure have been developed that exploit all the mechanisms we understand to be involved but they generally work on the slow system – this is why blood pressure changes following the introduction of anti-hypertensive drugs, or changes in their dosage, can take a few weeks to take full effect. Although this is not a complete account of blood pressure control – there are more hormones known to be important, for example – it is good enough for us to understand the logic behind the medical approach to hypertension.

Key Points

- The two main factors that determine blood pressure are the pumping action of the heart (cardiac output) and the width of the small arteries (arterioles) throughout the body (peripheral resistance).
- The body has several ways of controlling blood pressure, through the actions of the nervous system and various hormones that act on the heart and on the arterioles.
- The amount of salt (sodium) in the body is closely related to the level of blood pressure. Control of salt balance is therefore an essential part of blood pressure control.

Chapter 3

The Causes of Hypertension

With so much known about the biology of blood pressure it would be reasonable to assume we now understand what drives it up in people with hypertension, but not so. 95 per cent or more of people with hypertension do not have any demonstrable single 'fault' in the various mechanisms of blood pressure control. Of course we can surmise that hypertension relates in part to inefficiencies in these controls, but there is not usually one process we can identify and blame. This type of hypertension, termed 'essential' hypertension, is by far the most common and it's an unsatisfactory label – we still don't know the reasons for hypertension in the majority of people who have it.

Understanding hypertension completely is the aim of the large amount of research that continues into the condition. Our knowledge to date has however made it possible to design drugs that are effective against hypertension at many different stages of the blood pressure control system. These are covered in more detail in chapter 8.

Risk factors for essential hypertension

Although we do not yet know enough about why hypertension occurs, a number of 'risk factors' are known which increase the chance of it happening. Some of these, such as the amount of salt in our diet, are within our capability to change. Others, such as an inherited tendency to hypertension, we have to live with. One of the hopes of the present rapid advance in knowledge of genes and their behaviour is that this new understanding will reveal more reasons why hypertension occurs, and what we can do about it.

Modifiable risk factors

Four important modifiable risk factors for the development of essential hypertension are known:

- High dietary salt intake
- Low dietary potassium intake
- Excess body weight
- High alcohol intake.

SALT

The upwards drift in blood pressure with age, referred to in chapter 1, is seen only in individuals who eat a 'Western' style diet associated with a high intake of salt (i.e. sodium chloride). One of the largest population-based investigations of the effect of dietary salt on health was the Intersalt study. This involved over 10,000 individuals aged between 20 and 59 from 32 countries. It showed clearly that people who had a lower intake of salt had a significantly lower blood pressure than those with higher salt intakes (figure 9).

The Yi People Study in China compared Yi farmers in remote areas with those who had migrated to an urban area, and a group of Han residents of the same urban area. Blood pressure rose very little with age in the rural farmers but increased with age in the Yi migrants and

Figure 9: Effect of salt intake on blood pressure

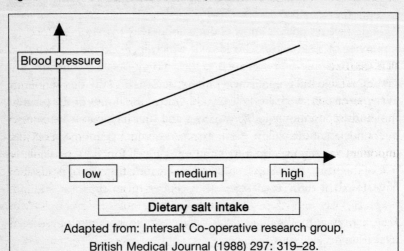

Adapted from: Intersalt Co-operative research group,
British Medical Journal (1988) 297: 319–28.

Han residents. Increased salt intake was one of the main identifiable differences in the rural and urban groups.

Reduction of dietary salt intake has been shown in several trials to lower blood pressure and appears to have the most effect on the blood pressure of elderly and black people – they are more 'salt sensitive'.

At around 10 grams daily, our intake of salt is two to three times greater than seems to be good for us. We should aim for a maximum intake of 5 grams of salt per day or less – a slightly heaped teaspoonful. There are several practical difficulties associated with trying to lower salt intake – extremely low salt diets taste unpalatable for a start, but food with tolerably reduced amounts of salt still take a little while to get used to. Although we can reduce the amount of salt we voluntarily add in cooking or at the table it is impossible to avoid the salt that is already in the food we buy. Hundreds of common foodstuffs have salt added during manufacture, so 70–80 per cent of the salt we eat is contained in processed food, including bread. Although the food industry is beginning to acknowledge the need for lowering salt it will be some time yet before low salt foods are the rule rather than the exception.

POTASSIUM

Common table salt contains sodium, but although it is the most abundant type of salt in the body it is neither the only one nor necessarily the most important. Other salts such as calcium have been mentioned in connection with muscle contraction. Potassium is another critically important salt involved in nerve and muscle cell function, particularly that of the heart. Population studies investigating the role of potassium have found it difficult to separate its effects from those of sodium, because potassium is present in fruit and vegetables, and people with a high fruit and vegetable intake tend also to have a low sodium intake. Increased potassium intake does however seem to be associated with less risk of hypertension. Potassium supplements are not recommended and for some people are potentially hazardous – for example those with impaired kidney function. The amount of potassium present in fruit and vegetables is enough to lower blood pressure so a boost of potassium is best achieved with a good daily intake of fruit, and not by taking potassium tablets or 'salt substitute' (potassium chloride).

BODY WEIGHT

Excess body weight is associated with hypertension. In chapter 4 we look at why overweight people may have their blood pressure measured incorrectly, but even when the pressure is accurately measured the association is seen. Weight loss lowers blood pressure but does so most effectively when accompanied by salt restriction. This illustrates the joined-up nature of risk factors – it is best to make some improvement in several areas rather than in only one.

ALCOHOL

Modest alcohol intake of around one half to two units daily appears to protect against the development of hardening of the arteries (atherosclerosis). (One unit of alcohol equals a standard glass of wine or a half pint of beer.) Higher intake of alcohol is associated with elevation of blood pressure, but the levels rapidly go down on removal of the alcohol. Alcohol consumption is probably not a cause of hypertension unless it is excessive and sustained.

STRESS

Sudden stress does cause blood pressure to rise but only temporarily. We tend to think of modern society as being 'stressful', and there is experimental evidence to show that people (mainly men) show their highest blood pressure levels during work. There is, however, as yet no clear evidence that stress in itself causes hypertension. This partly reflects the difficulty of measuring 'stress' – we use the word often but defining what we mean by it is very difficult. Having a 'stressful life' is by no means the sole province of the high-powered executive, as anyone struggling to get by on a low income will know very well. It makes common sense that when taking an overall approach to lifestyle factors one should attempt to make room for relaxation. In the short term this lowers blood pressure. The fact that we don't know for sure how stress fits in to the blood pressure picture does not mean that the experts think it is something to be ignored.

Attending a doctor's surgery is a common example of acute stress for many people, which has important implications for measuring blood pressure accurately (see 'White coat hypertension' in chapter 4).

Non-modifiable risk factors

AGE AND SEX

The increase in pressure with age is illustrated in figure 3 (see p 8). Between the ages of 35 and 60, systolic pressure goes up by an average of 20 mmHg and diastolic by about 10 mmHg. Women tend to have lower pressures than men until the menopause, when they start to catch men up, and at the elderly end of the range they have higher pressures than men. At all ages, those people with higher blood pressure have greater risk of cardiovascular problems than those of the same age but whose pressure is lower.

FAMILY HISTORY

High blood pressure tends to run in families although this probably accounts for only 25 per cent of the likelihood of developing hypertension. There are many possible factors that could account for this clustering. Families tend to eat the same sort of diet for example, and if this is high in salt and low in potassium then it could be this 'environment' in individuals who have an inherited tendency to hypertension that causes it to occur.

RACE

Hypertension is seen more commonly in black populations compared to whites but, as with family history, it's a mixed bag of possible explanations. The NHANES III population study in the USA showed significant differences between ethnic groups in the levels of blood pressure and in other important health-related features such as body weight, physical activity and likelihood of developing diabetes. There are important differences too between ethnic groups in their level of access to health care and education, particularly in the USA, but when these factors are taken into account the increased likelihood of hypertension remains. On the other hand hypertension is rare in rural areas of Africa and yet common in African city-dwellers. Again it seems that there are inheritable tendencies to hypertension, which in the right (or perhaps wrong) circumstances increase the chance of getting hypertension.

GENES

A small number of genetic changes have been identified in connection with some of the rarer causes of hypertension but these are outside the scope of this book. Examples include:

- Gordon's syndrome (raised blood pressure and blood potassium)
- Congenital adrenal hyperplasia (defect in natural steroid production due to absence or failure of one of several essential enzymes)
- Liddle's syndrome (over-activity of the sodium pump in the kidney, causing excess retention of sodium within the body, and loss of potassium).

As far as essential hypertension is concerned we can say that single gene defects are almost certainly not responsible, but that it is the interplay between many different genes and the environment that is important. This is an area of intense scientific research, and we should see some significant advances in our understanding of hypertension as a result within the next few years.

Uncommon causes of hypertension

Five per cent of people with hypertension have an identifiable, and possibly correctable, cause for the condition. It is therefore important to investigate hypertension properly when it is first noticed. The list of potentially responsible conditions is a long one but there are about half a dozen conditions that are reasonably easy to pick up and ought to be routinely looked for in any person newly diagnosed with hypertension. They fall under two main headings: kidney disorders and hormone disorders.

KIDNEY DISORDERS

The kidneys have a central role in regulating blood pressure and any disease affecting them can potentially disturb this function.

Impaired kidney blood supply

The cells within the kidneys that detect blood pressure and release renin can be 'fooled' if the arteries taking blood into the kidney are narrowed, because the blood will lose some of its pressure as it squeezes through the narrow artery. The blood reaching the kidney will therefore be at a low pressure, so the renin-producing cells will increase their output, sending the general blood pressure up inappropriately. The usual cause of such narrowing is the thickening of all arteries that comes with age, so it is usually not treatable but another, rare, cause is narrowing due to fibrous tissue within the walls of the blood vessel. This is more likely to be present in a young person with high blood pressure. Surgery to widen the artery can be done and if successful reverses the hypertension. This problem – called renal artery stenosis – can be present in one or both kidneys and should be looked for by scanners such as those that can detect blood flow within arteries deep in the body and by magnetic resonance scan (MRI) – a sophisticated scanning device which uses the body's response to magnetic fields to build up a detailed picture of internal structures.

Kidney tissue disease

A number of conditions are in this group, including glomerulonephritis (inflammation of the filtering system), diabetic kidney disease (see chapter 10), infection (usually the result of problems with the urine drainage tubes and bladder, allowing infection to spread up to the kidneys from below) and disorders known as connective tissue diseases which affect and damage arterioles, so reducing kidney blood flow. Blood and urine tests will give clues to the presence of these conditions.

Polycystic kidneys

This is a fairly rare condition that runs in families and causes fluid-filled bubbles (cysts) to form within kidney tissue. About a third of people with it also develop cysts in the liver. The cysts replace functioning kidney tissue and can cause kidney failure. Polycystic disease is sometimes not diagnosed until adulthood, by which time hypertension and some kidney damage has usually occurred. It can be detected by ultrasound scanning – which uses sound waves and their echoes or MRI scan.

HORMONE DISORDERS

Aldosterone

Overproduction of aldosterone by the adrenal glands causes too much retention of sodium and loss of potassium by the kidneys. In the rare condition called Conn's syndrome a tumour (usually benign and usually in one adrenal gland only) produces all of the excess aldosterone. The much more common condition – perhaps affecting as many as 10 per cent of hypertensive people – is that in which the general output of aldosterone by the adrenal glands is high. This is called 'idiopathic hyperaldosteronism', which literally means we don't know why it happens. A high level of aldosterone release from the adrenals can be suspected if a blood test shows high levels of sodium and low levels of potassium, so in someone with these blood findings and high blood pressure the aldosterone level should be measured. (The same blood results are seen in Liddle's syndrome, but further tests show the difference between the conditions.)

If investigation shows that there is a tumour producing the aldosterone (or more than one, as sometimes happens) the good news is that these tumours are usually not cancerous (they do not spread elsewhere in the body) and are removable by surgery. When the condition is due to general over-activity of the adrenal glands rather than a tumour it can be controlled partially or fully by the drug spironolactone, which blocks the effect of aldosterone (see chapter 8). In practice it may not be necessary for someone with an aldosterone-producing tumour to have it removed if his or her blood pressure is satisfactorily controlled on spironolactone treatment alone.

Adrenaline and noradrenaline

These are two similar chemical substances produced by the autonomic nervous system and tumours producing them can cause marked surges of blood pressure elevation accompanied by headaches, sweating attacks and a racing pulse. Most such tumours (called phaeochromocytomas) arise in the adrenal glands but other parts of the sympathetic nervous system can be the source. They are extremely rare but can be diagnosed by collecting the urine for 24 hours and analysing it for the presence of adrenaline-like substances. (This gets round the fact that the tumour secretes the hormone in bursts, so a single random urine sample might be negative if tested. Collecting the urine over a prolonged period catches the episodes of hormone output.) Surgical removal is the treatment of choice.

Cortisol

Cortisol is the main natural steroid of the body and once again is a product of the adrenal glands. Cushing's syndrome is the condition in which cortisol is produced in excess either by a tumour within the adrenal gland, or by over-stimulation of the adrenal gland by a tumour of the pituitary gland of the brain. The pituitary gland is a pea-sized gland connected to the underside of the brain and it has an importance that greatly exceeds its size. It acts like a master control centre, producing several different hormones, which control the activity of many other glands in the body. The thyroid gland, ovaries, testes and adrenal glands all take their orders from the pituitary gland through the signals it sends out, by the bloodstream, in the form of special hormones to which they are sensitive.

In the case of the adrenal glands this master hormone is ACTH (adrenocorticotrophic hormone). In Cushing's syndrome an ACTH-producing tumour of the pituitary gland stimulates the adrenals into overdrive. The features of Cushing's syndrome are similar to those of someone who has been on a high dose of steroid medication for a long time – hypertension, increased weight, puffy face, easy bruising of the skin and muscle and bone thinning.

Treatment of Cushing's syndrome is usually surgical – to the adrenal gland or the pituitary gland depending on the source of the problem. Cushing's syndrome is usually suspected from the person's appearance and confirmed by blood and urine tests of cortisol levels.

Key Points

1 The main 'modifiable' risk factors for developing hypertension are:
   - High dietary salt (sodium) intake
   - Low dietary potassium intake
   - Excess body weight
   - High alcohol intake
2 The main 'non-modifiable' risk factors are:
   - Age (blood pressure increases with age)
   - Sex (women have lower pressure than men until after the menopause)
   - Family history of hypertension
   - Race (hypertension is commoner in the black population)
3 95 per cent of people with hypertension have no identifiable cause for it. This is called 'essential' hypertension.
4 Hypertension should always be investigated to detect the small proportion of people whose blood pressure is raised because of another medical reason – 'secondary hypertension'.

Chapter 4

Practical Blood Pressure Measurement

History

The first scientific recording of blood pressure is credited to Reverend Stephen Hales in 1733. Hales (1677–1761) was one of those remarkable polymaths who made significant contributions to several branches of science, including the discovery of how plants raise water from their roots by the evaporation of water from their leaves. Using a sharpened goose quill as a hollow needle and the goose's windpipe as a flexible hose he '. . . caused a Mare to be tied down alive on her Back exposing an Artery in her upper Leg'. To the other end of the 'hose' he attached a vertical glass tube, showing that the pressure of the horse's blood 'caused it to rise in a column to a height of 8 feet 3 inches'.

For the modern, less invasive and more acceptable sphygmomanometer we have to thank an Italian doctor, Dr Scipione Riva-Rocci

(1863–1937). His invention of the mercury device around 1896 looks almost identical to the one still in use today. Although not the only sphygmomanometer that had been invented by then, the Riva-Rocci device was portable, accurate and gave consistent results. A Russian surgeon, Nicolai Sergeivich Korotkov (1874–1920), developed the system of measuring blood pressure by listening for sounds over an artery, in conjunction with a sphygmomanometer, in 1905.

Korotkov sounds

The Korotkov technique has been the standard in use throughout the world now for decades. He described five sounds, referred to as Phase 1 to 5 (or sometimes K1 to K5), that can be heard over an artery as a cuff above the artery has its pressure lowered from a value high enough to initially stop the blood coming through. What causes the Korotkov sounds is not fully understood but it relates to turbulence of blood flow within the artery being squeezed. In human beings the artery chosen is that in the front of the elbow – the 'brachial' artery – because it is easily heard by a stethoscope in this position and it is convenient to place the pressurised cuff around the upper arm.

When the cuff is inflated above the peak pumping pressure of the heart (the systolic pressure) the brachial artery is clamped shut, so no blood can come through and there is no sound. As the cuff pressure is lowered to equal and then drop below the systolic pressure, blood starts to come through the artery and is heard as a pulse with the stethoscope. This is Korotkov's first sound, or Phase 1. He described two other types of sound change just below the systolic pressure, calling them Phase 2 and 3 but they are unimportant and are ignored in ordinary medical practice. The next sound change, Phase 4, is heard as the pressure is dropped further and is a muffling of the sound of the pulse. When the cuff pressure is dropped a bit more the sound disappears, because the pressure on the artery is below that required to cause turbulence in the blood flow and hence any sound. Korotkov called the disappearance of sound Phase 5. The sounds and their significance are listed in table 1.

Table 1: Significance of Korotkov sounds

Korotkov Sound	Sound heard with stethoscope	Significance
Phase 1	Appearance of the pulse – a sharp, clear sound	Systolic blood pressure
Phase 2	Sound has a blowing or swishing quality	Not clinically significant
Phase 3	Sharp sound like Phase 1 but quieter	Not clinically significant
Phase 4	Sound becomes muffled	Diastolic pressure
Phase 5	Sound disappears	Diastolic pressure

Diastolic blood pressure is the low point that occurs just before the heart takes its next beat, and doctors have argued for a long time about whether the Phase 4 sound or the Phase 5 was the one which most accurately indicated diastolic pressure. For years it was more common to use Phase 4 sounds in the UK while the Americans preferred Phase 5. Debate has now settled in favour of Phase 5, with a couple of exceptions that are mentioned later in this book.

Apart from arguments over sounds there are some practical problems with the technique of measuring blood pressure in real life, which can potentially make enough differences to the readings to affect crucial decisions on diagnosis and treatment. We therefore need to go through them and understand how to minimise their effect.

Practical problems and solutions in blood pressure measurement

POSTURE

If we were to repeat Reverend Hales' eighteenth-century experiment with a modern probe that could safely check the pressure within any artery of the body we would see that blood pressure is not the same everywhere – for the simple reason that blood is heavy and gravity has its own effect. Imagine a cylinder of water (which is about the same density as blood) 2 metres high. The pressure within the water at the bottom is higher than that at the top because of the weight of water above it. The same is true of a person – blood pressure measured at the ankle in a standing person is higher than that at the top of the head.

The standard position, which has also been used in most of the research work on hypertension, has the person sitting, with his or her arm supported at the level of the heart – which is about half way down the breastbone (figure 10). A standard desk/chair combination in which the patient has to have his arm on the table will probably mean the arm is slightly too low – this can elevate the pressure artificially by 5–10 mmHg. A comfortable cushion should support the arm to the correct height or alternatively the doctor can support the patient's arm at the same time as he holds onto the stethoscope.

Figure 10: Correct position for blood pressure measurement

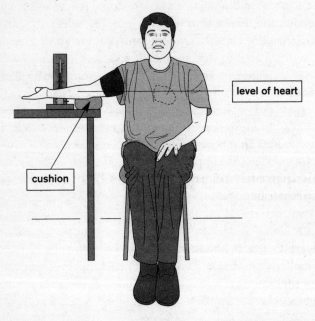

level of heart

cushion

An unsupported arm is useless for measuring blood pressure – the muscular action of keeping the arm up will raise the pressure considerably.

Electronic machines to measure blood pressure are now widely available for home use. These are covered shortly but at this point it is worth remembering that the same rule of checking the pressure at the level of the heart applies to them. A wrist-worn device will give very different readings depending on arm position.

Measuring blood pressure when the person is standing is valuable if it is suspected that a significant drop in blood pressure is occurring on standing up – for example if there is dizziness on rising. There are two main groups of people who suffer from this condition, called 'postural hypotension'. The first is elderly people on drug treatment for hypertension. The elderly have less ability to make the corrections to blood pressure that are required when standing and this is made worse by drug therapy. The second is people with diabetes, usually of long standing, who have as a result of the diabetes suffered some damage to the nervous system.

Small drops of pressure on standing, which are not accompanied by symptoms, can however be ignored.

SLEEVES

Sleeves of garments are often pushed up above the cuff as a means of saving time, but they are a menace. Not only does the bunched fabric prevent the cuff from being applied evenly and at the correct level across the muscle of the upper arm but also a tight sleeve will compress the underlying artery before it gets to the cuff. This will interfere with the Korotkov sounds and will make the reading inaccurate. A very loose-fitting half sleeve can probably be pushed out of the way without causing trouble, but the arm needs to be taken out of jumpers and long-sleeved shirts to take a proper reading.

NUMBER OF READINGS

Blood pressure is not a stable measurement and several readings need to be averaged before one can really say what the figure is. The British Hypertension Society's guidelines suggest that for someone with apparent mild hypertension and no other complications the average of two readings per visit at monthly intervals over four to six months should be taken before making a decision to treat. For someone getting a routine check two readings in the same arm about 30 seconds apart will suffice but if these differ by more than 5 mmHg further readings will be needed.

CUFF SIZE

Incorrect cuff size is a major source of incorrect readings. The purpose of the cuff is to efficiently squeeze the upper arm from all angles, so

Figure 11: Correct size of BP cuff

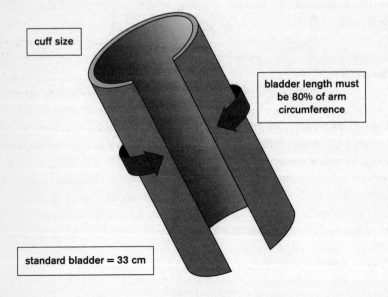

cuff size

bladder length must be 80% of arm circumference

standard bladder = 33 cm

it needs to circle the arm properly. Correct readings in fact require the long side of the bladder to be 80 per cent of the circumference of the arm (figure 11). Cuffs are made in two parts. The part you see is the outer cloth covering which has either a Velcro fastening or an extra length of cloth that can be wrapped around the arm and tucked in to keep it in position. The part that does the work is an oblong flat rubber bladder, which is connected to the tubing and enclosed within the cloth outer. Cuffs that are too small need to be pumped up harder to squeeze the arm effectively and so give falsely high readings. Cuffs that are too big can give falsely low readings for the opposite reason.

Many blood pressure cuffs in general use are too small – partly because historically the cuff size that was chosen as the standard was too small for many people but also because of the increased likelihood of a hypertensive person being overweight – and therefore having a thicker arm. The standard cuff has survived because virtually all research studies on hypertension have used it, but there is now a general trend to using larger cuffs. Many doctors now use the 'alternative adult cuff', which is slightly bigger than the standard cuff and more suitable for the British population. Even better would be an adjustable cuff that always fits – these are being developed.

The standard cuff is suitable for an adult with an arm circumference of 33 cm or less. The alternative adult cuff will suit an arm up to 42 cm. Bigger arms need bigger cuffs.

INSTRUMENT PROBLEMS

The beauty of the mercury column is that it depends only on gravity to work, whereas most aneroid (air pressure) machines contain pressure-sensitive diaphragms, gear wheels and levers – so are more prone to mechanical errors. Both types of machine can have leaky tubes or bladders, dodgy valves and tired out Velcro fastenings with poor grip, all of which cause inaccuracies. Mercury's days are numbered, at least as far as general use is concerned, but many research workers in the field of hypertension will probably continue to use mercury machines because of their reliable accuracy.

Having a mercury manometer is however no guarantee on its own that the instrument is accurate. In a survey of one inner city primary care group 2.3 per cent of mercury and 14.8 per cent of aneroid sphygmomanometers failed accuracy tests. There is no national standard regulating the quality and accuracy of these machines – it is entirely up to the practice or hospital whether they are calibrated or maintained properly.

ELECTRONIC DEVICES
Electronic blood pressure measuring devices have been around since at least the 1980s but their acceptance has been slow until the past few years because of a lack of faith in their accuracy. With the mercury device heading for extinction and the fact that at least some electronic sphygmomanometers are now clearly able to measure blood pressure accurately they are set to become the dominant means of testing blood pressure within the near future.

In many situations they are already the norm because they offer a number of potential advantages. They avoid some of the errors of interpretation that humans are prone to make, they are environmentally friendly, portable, getting cheaper all the time, can memorise multiple readings and can be connected to computers to produce useful data outputs. The accuracy of the machines depends on the quality of design and build and the robustness of the software within the electronics. These are now of a very high standard and further details on the procedures used to check the accuracy of electronic devices, and which devices are capable of meeting such standards, are at the end of this chapter.

No machine is, however, completely reliable – they still have to be checked periodically and maintained properly. There is a range of quality and accuracy – you get what you pay for. Above all there is the fact that electronic manometers are relatively new to the blood pressure scene. Almost all of the medical research done on blood pressure over the past several decades has been done with the Riva-Rocci type mercury manometer. Very little of the information in the established medical literature has been obtained with electronic machines – and we do not yet know if the data obtained in the older studies is automatically valid for the newer methods. This is largely because the potential sources of error and bias in the 'old method', where a human reads the blood pressure, are different to those that apply to machine readers. I've covered some of those points in the first part of this chapter – let's now look at the other important sources of error.

Human sources of error in blood pressure measurement

THE OBSERVER

Hearing

In the standard method of blood pressure measurement the doctor or nurse listens for the sounds of blood flowing in an arm, using a stethoscope. Clearly those observers whose hearing is less than perfect could have difficulty hearing the sounds. Such a difficulty will under-estimate the systolic pressure (because the first few beats may be quieter) and overestimate the diastolic pressure (because one is listening for the disappearance of sound, which will occur earlier for a partially deaf person). Good quality stethoscopes help, and they are not very expensive, but many cheap stethoscopes with poor acoustic performance are still in use in surgeries, out-patient clinics and hospital wards. Amplified stethoscopes are available for those with particular hearing difficulty but the electronic sphygmomanometer is a better solution, using sensors to detect the pressure, which are independent of the observer's hearing ability.

Haste

Doctors and nurses are busy folk and not immune to taking shortcuts under pressure of time. Getting the patient's arm properly exposed out of the sleeve is often bypassed. Taking one measurement rather than several with time between for the patient to relax is often done and is inadequate when making critical readings. Worst perhaps is the 'quickie' reading – when the whole procedure is done too quickly to be accurate. Dropping the cuff pressure too fast has the same error-producing potential as the observer with poor hearing. If the pressure is allowed to fall quickly then in the time between two heartbeats it may have fallen several millimetres below the true systolic pressure. The diastolic pressure is recorded when the last beat is heard but this might not be the lowest pressure beat that could have been heard had more time been taken. The result is a reading that is lower than the correct systolic and higher than the correct diastolic.

Guidelines of The British Hypertension Society and American Heart Association state that the cuff should be blown up to 20–30 mmHg above the systolic pressure and then allowed to fall by 2 mm per second. So someone with a normal pressure of 120/70 mmHg should take at least half a minute to read. Skilful observers can make an accurate reading a little more quickly by accelerating the drop between Phase 1 and Phase 4 but beware the ten-second pressure check – it could be wildly inaccurate. Electronic manometers go at a fixed speed and avoid this problem. They also free the doctor or nurse to get on with something else while it goes about its work, so lessening the time pressure on the professional.

Observer position

When reading a mercury sphygmomanometer the observer's eye needs to be level with the top of the mercury column, for reasons illustrated in figure 12. The effect has been exaggerated here to show the principle but if the observer looks at the column from above, he'll see a falsely low reading and from too low an angle the reading will be falsely high. In practice errors of +/- 2 mmHg can occur from this mistake. Air pressure (aneroid) sphygmomanometers tend to have clock face dials, which do not have this type of error.

Terminal digit preference

A grand-sounding term for the fact that doctors, who are human, round off the pressure reading to a 'preferred' reading – usually either zero or 5. The scale on sphygmomanometers is marked off in one or two

Figure 12: Effect of eye level on reading a mercury column

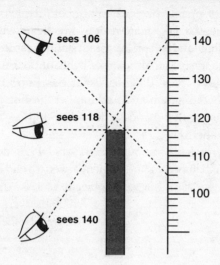

millimetre divisions and the pressure should be recorded to the nearest mark above the observed reading. In practice, doctors are many times more likely to record a reading with a zero in its ending like, for example, 130 mm rather than 133 mm, which might have been the actual reading.

Decision bias

This is another uniquely human type of error that, like terminal digit preference, can be eliminated by machine measurement. Essentially it means that the doctor has made up his mind (perhaps quite subconsciously) what the blood pressure will be before he has measured it. For example a young man with previously normal readings shows a mildly raised pressure on a random check but as he seems excessively anxious in the surgery that day the doctor rounds the reading down to something more 'normal'. Or an overweight lady already on three different anti-hypertensive drugs attends for a check-up on a busy Friday night when both she and the doctor are tired and the waiting room is still full of people overdue to be seen. Her blood pressure is just as high as at the last examination, but the doctor accepts it's probably just 'stress' and keeps the treatment the same. In both cases there has been a decision in advance – in one case the doctor is reluctant to make a new diagnosis that has important long-term implications in a young man and in the other the doctor has decided that the battle against this particular lady's blood pressure is one that he'll defer to another day.

This type of error is serious but hard to avoid when dealing with the reality of human behaviour. It is much better to eliminate it with a device that has no choice but to be objective.

THE PATIENT

'White coat hypertension'

It has been known for years that patients have lower blood pressures when they measure it themselves or when they have it measured by nurses rather than doctors. The 'white coat effect' can occur with the most apparently relaxed of patients and occurs even when the doctor doesn't wear a white coat! Temporary elevations of as much as 30 mmHg can be seen in people who demonstrate this effect, which is of course more than enough to give a completely inaccurate picture of someone's true blood pressure. The white coat effect occurs in 15–30 per cent of the general population, including those who have perfectly normal blood pressure and those who have genuine hypertension. Detecting white coat hypertension can be of major importance, particularly when making the diagnosis of hypertension and in monitoring the effect of treatment.

White coat hypertension should be suspected if:

• There is a considerable drop in blood pressure between the start and end of a clinic attendance (some drop in blood pressure is

normal as the person becomes more relaxed, and this fall is more pronounced in 'white coat hypertensives').
• There is variation between readings taken by the doctor and, say, the practice nurse.
• There is variation between readings taken at the surgery and at home – best made with an electronic sphygmomanometer. (In fact this variability between home and clinic readings when every other factor is the same is the definition of white coat hypertension!)

White coat hypertension is important for reasons other than causing confusion when measuring blood pressure readings:

1 There is some evidence to suggest that people with white coat hypertension are more prone to develop features of true hypertension, such as thickening of the heart muscle over time. The evidence is not yet clear, but white coat hypertension should be regarded as a reason for regular blood pressure checks even if it is not high enough to merit treatment.
2 Hypertensive people with a tendency to show the white coat effect will seem to have higher blood pressures when they attend the GP's surgery, which will in turn make it likely for them to be over-treated with anti-hypertensive medication. Outside the surgery the effect of the drugs can make their pressure fall too low i.e. they become hypotensive. This might be suspected if the person experiences light-headedness on standing up or excessive fatigue on treatment.

The preferred technique to detect the white coat effect is ambulatory blood pressure measurement.

Ambulatory blood pressure measurement

BASIC TECHNIQUE AND APPLICATION
Portable machines capable of taking repeated blood pressure measurements over a prolonged period (usually 24 hours) have been around

since the 1960s. As the size of modern electronic devices continues to fall and the need for us to define hypertension more accurately increases we will see more use of ambulatory blood pressure measurement (ABPM). The equipment consists of a standard-looking blood pressure cuff connected to an automatic, battery-powered pump and measuring unit that is about the size of a small book and is worn around the belt. Left to itself the device will trigger periodically (typically every 15 to 30 minutes) and take a blood pressure reading while the wearer goes about his or her business, including sleep. During sleep the readings are taken less often – every 30 to 60 minutes usually. The information is recorded on a chip inside the control unit and can be fed into a computer for analysis at the end of the measuring period.

ABPM machines need to be light enough to wear comfortably, robust enough to take the ordinary jostling around of a person on the move and accurate enough to give consistent results. They cost several thousand pounds, require regular maintenance and skill in their application and the results need expert interpretation. As yet therefore, ABPM is not a technique that has been widely taken up at the level of the general practitioner. All GPs in the UK should however have access to a regional centre, under the management of a consultant in hypertension medicine, which can offer an ABPM service when required.

ABPM measurement can be useful when:

- White coat hypertension is suspected
- Blood pressure readings vary a lot from reading to reading
- Blood pressure appears difficult to control, despite the use of multiple drugs.

ABPM could be more widely used within general practice if more manpower and funding resources became available. Perhaps 20 per cent of people currently taking blood pressure treatment are being 'over-treated' because they actually have white coat hypertension and ABPM could help identify them, allowing their treatment to be withdrawn. This would considerably benefit the patients as well as the health care system, but we need to wait a bit longer until research information indicates more precisely the role of ABPM in practice.

Table 2: Upper limits of 'normal' blood pressures in ambulatory blood pressure monitoring

	Systolic pressure (mmHg)	Diastolic pressure (mmHg)
Daytime	135	85
Night-time	120	70

PATTERNS OF BLOOD PRESSURE SEEN IN ABPM

In all people the levels of blood pressure seen in ABPM are lower than those obtained in static measurements. The differences are in the region of 10–20 mmHg in systolic pressure and 5–10 mmHg in diastolic readings, which are quite large figures in the field of blood pressure. Hence lower thresholds for normal blood pressures are generally accepted, as shown in table 2. These figures also reflect the fact that blood pressure tends to fall during sleep.

Most people with hypertension also show this 'dip' of blood pressure during sleep but ABPM reveals a smaller group of people with hypertension who do not. They are called 'non-dippers' and there is some evidence to suggest that these people are at higher risk of developing the problems associated with prolonged hypertension. This could be because the proportion of the time per 24 hours that their blood pressure is elevated is greater than 'dippers'. The medical jargon term for this concept is 'cardiovascular load' i.e. the more time the blood pressure is high, the greater is the cardiovascular load.

Home-based blood pressure monitoring

The availability of reliable electronic sphygmomanometers at reasonable cost has opened up the possibility of people checking their own blood pressures at home. This is a compromise between ambulatory monitoring and entirely clinic-based readings and offers a number of advantages, but some disadvantages.

The white coat effect is eliminated and a number of readings can be taken over a period of days or weeks, giving a better overall picture of the person's blood pressure. As these machines are more affordable than ambulatory ones there is more scope for home monitors to be used within general practice. The involvement of the individual with his or her own blood pressure measurement is a considerable advantage, allowing more scope for dialogue between the person and the doctor or nurse. Home measurement can be very reassuring if it shows lower (or even normal readings) when clinic readings have been high or borderline.

Disadvantages include the need for good training of both patient and doctor in the technique and interpretation of results. As with ABPM and electronic blood pressure measurement in general we are still 'finding our feet' concerning how best to use home monitors, but they appear very helpful in judging the size of the white coat effect and look set to be used increasingly often.

Accuracy of electronic sphygmomanometers

Any measuring device has to be accurate and reliable, and there are two published standards against which blood pressure monitors can be judged – those of the British Hypertension Society (BHS) and the American Association for the Advancement of Medical Instrumentation (AAMI). Information on machines that meet the necessary standards has been summarised by a working group from the European Society of Hypertension in the British Medical Journal at http://bmj.com/cgi/content/full/322/7285/531. This list is based on published literature and is neither exhaustive nor a guarantee that any particular machine will be better than another, but as the number of machines increases it makes sense to check that they have satisfied the BHS and/or the AAMI standards before purchase. Devices with arm cuffs (rather than wrist or finger cuffs) are preferred. At the time of writing (January 2002) the following automatic (i.e. self-inflating) machines are recommended for use:

- Omron HEM-705 CP   (Omron Healthcare Ltd)
- Omron HEM-722C
- Omron HEM-735C
- Omron HEM-713C
- Omron HEM-737 Intellisense.
  (Source: O'Brien, British Medical Journal, 2001 – see appendix A)

This list represents only a tiny fraction of the number of available devices, and will grow as more are assessed and passed. Details of other monitors that have been tested can be obtained from the distributors (see appendix C for contact details).

As with ABPM, lower values for the upper limit of normal blood pressure are accepted for home monitoring: 135 mmHg for systolic pressure and 85 mmHg for diastolic pressure.

Key Points

- Accurate blood pressure measurement requires good instruments, good technique, and a relaxed patient.
- Many sources of error can easily make blood pressure readings inaccurate.
- Several readings are needed at different times to make a proper estimation of someone's blood pressure.
- Electronic BP measuring machines are becoming increasingly popular and available for both professional and home use.
- The 'white coat effect' is a significant cause of over-estimation of someone's blood pressure.

Chapter 5

Your Blood Pressure

Chapter 4 illustrated that blood pressure measurement, although simple in concept, needs to be done properly if it is to be accurate. The technique, equipment and circumstances are all important. Getting your own blood pressure checked properly is very important to your health, and there is a lot you can do to ensure that it happens as it should.

Tips for accurate blood pressure checks

GET IT CHECKED!

The first thing is to think – when did I last have my blood pressure measured? According to the British Hypertension Society every adult should have a check every five years at least. High blood pressure is a condition that causes no symptoms in the early stages and you should certainly make an appointment with your doctor or practice nurse if this length of time has elapsed since you were last seen. Many doctors feel a shorter gap of around three years is preferable between routine checks if the readings are normal. Don't wait for your doctor to send an appointment reminding you to come along. Many practices will do this but the pressure on GPs is too high for even the best-organised practices to ensure that everyone who needs to be seen is called up.

If your practice is always closed by the time you get home from work enquire if they have Saturday appointments or a late evening surgery to accommodate you. Get it checked during a holiday break if you have to, or enquire if your employer has an occupational health service.

MEASURE YOUR ARM SIZE

The alternative adult cuff is suitable for an adult whose upper arm does not exceed 42 cm circumference. Before you go along to the surgery, measure your arm circumference with a tape measure. If you have a big arm, you will need a big cuff. Enquire which size of cuff is being used if you are unsure, and insist upon the correct one.

GET YOUR SLEEVE OFF

A bunched up sleeve from a shirt, blouse or jumper above a blood pressure cuff is useless. Don't wait to be asked to get your arm properly exposed – do it anyway. A loose-fitting half-sleeve shirt or T-shirt will probably be all right to just move out of the way so long as it doesn't feel tight.

BE AWARE OF GOOD (AND BAD) TECHNIQUE

Health professionals can be under a lot of time pressure but sloppy technique is never justifiable. You should be seated comfortably, with your arm supported so that your elbow is about level with your heart (figure 10, see p 46) and your palm is facing upwards. This will mean a cushion is required under your arm if the doctor's desk is too low. Ask for one if it isn't offered.

The preferred position for blood pressure measurement is sitting. You can have your pressure checked while lying down, which might help reduce the white coat effect if you feel very keyed up while having the reading taken. Provided the arm is supported at heart height lying down does not influence the true blood pressure reading significantly but almost all guidelines in hypertension are based on measurements on the seated person.

The tubing of the cuff is best arranged so it comes in at the upper edge (shoulder side – see figure 2) rather than the lower edge. Many doctors and nurses are used to connecting it the latter way round, which with many cuffs places the tubes exactly where the stethoscope is supposed to go. Some cuffs have a printed mark or arrow that should line up with the middle of the hollow of the elbow (the position of the artery). If there is such a mark and it is not lined up properly then the cuff is in the wrong place.

If, when the pressure is pumped up, the Velcro of the cuff starts to tear itself apart then the cuff is useless. Any reading taken with such a cuff should be disregarded. It is not acceptable for an old Velcro cuff to be held together by the doctor or nurse while the blood pressure is being taken – this distorts the pressure on the arm.

The person taking your blood pressure should, if using a mercury sphygmomanometer, get their eye to the same level as the top of the mercury column (figure 12, see p 53).

The pressure should be increased quickly to about 30 mmHg above your systolic pressure and then let down by about 2 mm per second (electronic machines do this part automatically). With a mercury or aneroid instrument see if you can watch the reading during the measurement – if it falls very much more quickly than 2 mm per second then the reading's accuracy will be doubtful.

There is one other check you can do, which again depends on you being able to see the reading during the procedure. When the cuff is pumped up higher than your systolic blood pressure there is no blood flowing in your arm. You will notice at this point that you cannot feel any pulse in your arm. As the cuff pressure falls and eventually is equalled by your systolic blood pressure you will begin to feel a pulse beat – under the cuff – as the blood begins to flow through. This is not very easy to do and it can be misleading, but if there is a large difference between the pressure at which you begin to feel the blood flowing back into your arm and what the doctor or nurse says is your systolic blood pressure, then you should raise the matter with them. You cannot detect your own diastolic blood pressure by this method however.

If every reading that you get on a blood pressure check seems to end in a zero (or perhaps a 5) this will suggest terminal digit preference on the part of the observer. Blood pressure varies in all of us and it is equally likely to end in any 1 mm step between zero and 9.

GET SEVERAL READINGS
One blood pressure measurement is never enough. In any one session at least two readings are better than one and when deciding upon borderline hypertension then two readings per month for four to six months should be taken before deciding. It is useful to alter the time of blood pressure checks, so as to get a better impression of how it varies during the day.

Standards of care

The preceding points may sound like nit picking and many health professionals might take offence at the suggestion they take anything other than the utmost care when measuring blood pressure. The evidence suggests, however, that standards of care in blood pressure management are not as good as they should be, and these quality points should be seen as essential ingredients of good care.

Many people would feel uncomfortable saying to their doctor or nurse that they felt their blood pressure had been taken incorrectly. This book will not turn anyone into a hypertension expert, but no health professional should mind if a patient raises an issue of importance to his or her health even if initially it might seem critical. The purpose of this book is to encourage dialogue between doctor and patient, on the basis of an adequate degree of knowledge on the part of both.

Action levels for blood pressure (measured within 'surgery setting' and based on British Hypertension Society Guidelines 1999)

Normal
- Systolic pressure consistently below 135 mmHg is normal, and consistently below 120 mmHg is considered ideal
- Diastolic pressure consistently below 85 mmHg is normal, and consistently below 80 mmHg is considered ideal

Action: re-check every 5 years until 80 years old

'High normal'
- Systolic pressure between 135 and 139 mmHg
- Diastolic pressure between 85 and 90 mmHg

Action: repeat blood pressure checks annually

Borderline
- Systolic pressure between 140 and 159 mmHg
- Diastolic pressure between 90 and 99 mmHg

Action: two groups of people require different actions:

1 Group 1 (*any one or more of these qualifies*):
   - Any evidence of blood pressure damage to tissues like kidneys or heart
   - Presence of diabetes
   - Calculated 'cardiovascular risk' above 15 per cent over the next 10 years (explained in chapter 7)

Action: lower the blood pressure with treatment

2 Group 2 (*need all three to qualify*)
  • Not diabetic
  • No evidence of blood pressure damage to tissues
  • Cardiovascular risk below 15 per cent over the next 10 years

Action: no treatment but observe annually

Hypertensive
• Systolic pressures greater or equal to 160 mmHg
• Diastolic pressures greater or equal to 100 mmHg

Action: elevation of *either* systolic or diastolic pressure to these levels requires treatment

Important note: Systolic and diastolic pressures are independent of each other – only one needs to be too high, not both, to merit treatment (see chapter 9 for a discussion on the importance of raised systolic but normal diastolic pressure).

Thresholds and targets

The preceding figures are the 'thresholds' of blood pressure at which action is triggered in various circumstances. Once a decision is made that someone has hypertension, and that treatment is necessary, one then needs a target to aim for. One might say that achieving a normal blood pressure (less than 135/85 or even 120/80) should be the aim and indeed if that can be done then well and good. In practice, however, such rigorous targets are hard to attain and it is better to choose one that is a) likely to be achievable and b) makes a significantly good improvement in cardiovascular risk. The currently recommended *target* blood pressure for hypertensive people on treatment is less than 140/85 mmHg (British Hypertension Society).

DIABETES

Diabetes is a special case. People with diabetes are less able to handle sugar (glucose) within the body due to inefficiency or lack of the hormone insulin. Diabetes developing in younger people usually needs to be treated with insulin injections whereas diabetes in older people can be treated with tablets or, if very mild, with diet alone.

One of the problems associated with longstanding diabetes is the development of hardening of the arteries and increased risk of stroke, heart attack and kidney damage. The chance of this occurring can be reduced by good control of the diabetes and also by strict blood pressure control. As a result, the targets for high blood pressure control in diabetes (of all types) are tougher than for non-diabetic people and are currently set at less than 140/80 mmHg (British Hypertension Society).

Deciding to treat

When clinic blood pressures are high but white coat hypertension is suspected of raising it, or when blood pressure elevation is modest and a decision to treat is difficult, then the extra measures such as ambulatory or home-based measurements need to be considered to clarify whether hypertension is really present, and to what degree.

There is an important exception to this – when there is already evidence of tissue damage from hypertension or when the calculated cardiovascular risk is above 15 per cent over the next ten years. Here the need for treatment is already established, and it should be commenced without further delay. In such a person clinic blood pressure levels are adequate to guide treatment decisions.

Key Points

- Hypertension is under-diagnosed. It is important for all adults to ensure they have their blood pressure checked periodically, so if yours hasn't been done for a while, make a date to have it done at your GP's surgery.
- Blood pressure of less than 135/85 mm/Hg is normal and below 120/80 mmHg is ideal.
- 'High normal' is between 135 and 139 systolic and between 85 and 90 diastolic. It needs watching annually but does not need treatment in the absence of any other risk factors.
- Everyone with blood pressure over 140/90 mmHg needs either treatment or careful watching, depending on other risk factors. For people with diabetes the threshold is 140/80 mm/Hg.
- Everyone with blood pressure over 160/100 mmHg needs treatment.
- Systolic and diastolic blood pressures are equally important. Raised level of either merits the same action as listed above for both.

Chapter 6

The Investigation of High Blood Pressure

In chapter 3 the possible causes of hypertension were outlined, noting that in only around 5 per cent of people newly diagnosed with hypertension will an identifiable cause be found. It is essential nonetheless that hypertension is properly investigated and correctable causes sought.

History

Any medical assessment properly starts with questions concerning symptoms, which will hardly ever be fruitful in hypertension – it is a symptomless condition. Headaches and nosebleeds are popularly thought to indicate high blood pressure, and indeed a small number of people with hypertension do experience headaches, but you really can't tell what your blood pressure is until someone measures it properly. In the very rare condition of an adrenaline-producing tumour (phaeochromocytoma) blood pressures can peak very high and cause headaches along with sweating attacks and a racing pulse.

A family tendency to hypertension will be relevant to note but does not give any clue to the cause of hypertension. Diabetes should always be looked for by investigation, but a family history of it will increase the chance of it being present. At this point it is very useful to go over lifestyle factors that are relevant to hypertension – those which are known either to increase the likelihood of hypertension occurring (raised dietary salt and alcohol intake and being overweight) or which are relevant to cardiovascular risk (dietary fat intake, smoking and exercise habit). Breathlessness or chest pain on effort might indicate that the heart is already struggling to cope and pains in the legs on walking can suggest hardening of the arteries to the leg muscles. These are late features of hypertension – by detecting high blood pressure early and taking effective corrective action these complications should be avoided.

A small number of medications can increase blood pressure or potentially interfere with anti-hypertensive medicines and should be noted. Examples include non-steroidal anti-inflammatory drugs (NSAIDs) such as ibuprofen, which are commonly used as painkillers, and steroid therapy. The oral contraceptive pill causes reversible hypertension in a small proportion of women. Every medical student learns that liquorice addiction causes hypertension and spends the rest of his or her life looking for someone with it – but it does occur.

Appearance

Some conditions, such as Cushing's syndrome in which the body's natural steroid production is overactive, can cause characteristic changes in appearance that a doctor will recognise. Cushing's syndrome is rare – a general practitioner might see one person with it in his professional lifetime compared to many dozens if not hundreds of people with essential hypertension.

Body weight

Excess body weight is associated with hypertension, and with increased risk of cardiovascular disease. Weight and height are related and knowledge of both is needed before one can say if a person is overweight. A simple mathematical formula relating the two is now universally used to do this – the Body Mass Index (BMI). To calculate a BMI, take the person's weight (in kilograms) and divide it by the square of their height (in metres). For example, an 80 kg person of height 1.7 m will have a BMI of $80/(1.7 \times 1.7) = 27.7$ kg/m^2 (the BMI formula applies equally to men and women). The ranges of BMI are:

- Normal   =   20-24.9
- Overweight =   25-30
- Obese   =   Over 30

Table 3 shows a range of heights and the associated weights for the normal and obese ranges.

Clinical examination

General clinical examination in someone with essential hypertension will be normal unless hypertension has already been present long enough to cause tissue or organ effects such as:

- Enlargement of the heart – which can be judged more easily in a thin person and shows as a heave under the left ribs with each heartbeat.
- Narrowing of leg arteries – the pulses in one or both feet and legs will be reduced.
- Changes to the blood vessels at the back of the eye. These start as subtle variations of the width of the blood vessels and eventually (usually years later) show as small bleeds and leakage areas.

Otherwise examination will perhaps pick up only the rarer causes of hypertension:

Table 3: Body mass index guide

| Height (less shoes) | | | Weight range (kg) | Obese weight (kg) |
Metres	Feet	Inches	for BMI 20–24.9	for BMI >30
1.50	4	11	45–56	68
1.52	5	0	46–58	69
1.54	5	1	47–59	71
1.56	5	1	49–61	73
1.58	5	2	50–62	75
1.60	5	3	51–64	77
1.62	5	4	52–66	79
1.64	5	5	53–67	81
1.66	5	5	55–69	83
1.68	5	6	56–71	85
1.70	5	7	58–72	87
1.72	5	8	59–74	89
1.74	5	8	61–75	91
1.76	5	9	62–77	93
1.78	5	10	63–79	95
1.80	5	11	65–81	97
1.82	6	0	66–83	99
1.84	6	0	68–85	102
1.86	6	1	69–86	104
1.88	6	2	71–88	106
1.90	6	3	72–90	108

- Swelling of the kidneys and/or liver in polycystic disease.
- Delay in the pulse reaching the groin artery compared with the pulse at the wrist. (Normally the pulse arrives at these points simultaneously as they are equally distant from the heart. In the rare condition of 'coarctation of the aorta' there is a narrow band within the part of the aorta 'downstream' of the major artery branches to

the arms and head. This causes high blood pressure in the arms and upper half of the body, and reduced pressure in the lower half. It can be corrected by surgery. It is very unusual for this condition to be diagnosed in adulthood – it is usually detected in infancy.)

ELECTROCARDIOGRAM

A tracing of the electrical activity of the heart – an electrocardiogram (ECG) – gives very useful information and should now be considered routine for all newly diagnosed hypertensive people. Many GPs have an ECG machine in the surgery but all will have access to the facility via the local hospital. Taking an ECG is painless, easy and quick. Wires are clipped to each wrist and ankle, and another is placed in different positions across the front of the chest. Most modern ECG machines are automatic and complete the test in a few minutes. The ECG tracing gives a good indication of the size of the heart muscle, which in turn indicates if the heart is working under excessive load.

Everyone newly diagnosed with hypertension should have an ECG, but there is a good case for doing the test also in many people being treated for hypertension. Sometimes it will make little or no difference to the treatment – for example someone with poor leg circulation and high blood pressure needs the pressure reduced to the target level no matter what the ECG indicates. But if someone with no obvious hypertension damage and whose blood pressure is slightly high has an ECG indicating some heart strain then this should increase efforts to get the pressure to target level or below.

The ECG provides a record that can be used for comparison in later years to judge if heart strain is getting better or worse. Occasionally it will reveal signs of reduced blood supply to the heart in someone who does not yet have any symptoms of it, i.e. angina, or chest pain on effort.

CHEST X-RAY

This is only useful to confirm if the heart is enlarged, or to investigate breathlessness. Normally a chest X-ray is of no value in assessing hypertension and is unnecessary.

URINE TESTS

Modern 'test strips' allow multiple urine tests to be done easily and quickly – about one minute is all it takes. Each plastic strip has a number of small coloured test squares stuck to it, each capable of doing a different test once dipped in urine – the square changes colour according to the result of the test.

The most useful urine strip tests are for:

- Protein or blood – if present suggests kidney disease.
- Glucose – if present suggests diabetes. Diabetes does not always show on urine tests however and must be checked with a blood test. Diabetes does not cause hypertension but if present the complications of hypertension can be more severe, and blood pressure control in diabetes needs to be particularly good.

Twenty-four-hour collections of urine are needed to diagnose phaeo-chromocytoma – by looking for excess adrenaline-like substances, but this is an exceptionally rare cause of hypertension. Not essential but nonetheless helpful is a 24-hour urine collection analysed for sodium and potassium, the output of which relates to the amounts we take in our diet. This can make it very clear how much salt comes to us in processed foods.

BLOOD TESTS

- Kidney function is assessed from the blood levels of normal bypro-ducts of the body's metabolism – the substances 'urea' and 'creatinine'. Both levels increase when kidney function drops.

- High sodium and low potassium levels suggest excess aldosterone production (chapter 3).
- Raised liver enzymes may suggest excess alcohol intake.
- Blood glucose levels will diagnose or exclude diabetes.
- Blood cholesterol, like glucose, will help in the overall assessment of cardiovascular risk.

These tests can all be done on a single sample of blood.

FURTHER INVESTIGATION

All of the preceding tests can and should be carried out by the general practitioner. If underlying conditions such as excess aldosterone production and other hormone disturbances, renal artery narrowing, polycystic kidney disease or any other complicating condition is suspected then a specialist's help will also be required. This will either be a physician with a special interest in hypertension, or a specialist in hormone disturbance (endocrinologist). People with exceptionally high blood pressure or who already show significant hypertensive tissue damage at diagnosis will also be likely to benefit from the expertise of the specialist in hypertension. However, the majority of people will be perfectly adequately assessed and treated by the general practitioner alone.

Key Points

- The majority of people with hypertension can be adequately investigated (and treated) by their general practitioner.
- A specialist in hypertension is used when an underlying cause for hypertension is suspected or when a person's blood pressure proves difficult to control.

Chapter 7

Estimating Health Risks

High blood pressure occurs in people, and people are complex. Treating the blood pressure reading without looking at the whole person is like checking a car's tyres now and again but neglecting every other aspect of vehicle maintenance. It is a valid criticism of modern medicine that we have become very drug oriented. High blood pressure treatment has too often been regarded in the light of which drug to use at the expense of lifestyle factors, which are very important but unfortunately are a lot harder to tackle. In chapter 1 we looked at how important is the interaction between many different aspects of an individual's makeup – age, sex, blood pressure, body weight, cholesterol level, smoking history, family history and presence or absence of diabetes – which all have effects upon the ultimate risk of developing hardening of the arteries, heart attack or stroke – the 'cardiovascular risk'.

Risk calculators

We now know enough about the relative importance of various factors to put some figures on them and estimate an individual's chance of a major event such as a heart attack or stroke occurring over the following five or ten years. Such an exercise is particularly useful to show how changing some of the modifiable risk factors, such as smoking or high blood pressure, can have a marked effect upon an individual's risk. A number of tools exist which allow you to do this for yourself or with the help of your doctor or practice nurse. Some use computer programs, and others can be done with pen and paper. The self-assessment that follows (tables 4 and 5) is derived from that published by Pocock and colleagues (see appendix A). It is also available as both an online test and a free computer program on the internet at www.riskscore.org.uk.

You need the following information to complete the test, some of which you will need to ask your doctor to provide from your medical records:

1 Age and sex
2 Height (metres)
3 Systolic blood pressure (an average of the last three readings from your GP will do)
4 Total cholesterol concentration in the blood (in millimoles per litre – written as mmol/l – the standard units used in the UK)
5 Smoking history – count yourself as a smoker if you have smoked any amount regularly during the past two years
6 Presence or absence of diabetes (whether diet-controlled, diet and tablets, or insulin-dependent)
7 Whether you have previously had a stroke or a heart attack
8 Creatinine concentration in the blood (in micromoles per litre – written as µmol/l – also the standard units used in the UK)
9 Whether you have been diagnosed to have thickened heart muscle (the medical term is 'left ventricular hypertrophy' and the evidence for it would be present in an electrocardiogram test).

Table 4: Cardiovascular risk assessment (women)

For each row, choose the 'Risk Points' figure which corresponds with your own details and write it in the right hand 'Risk Score' column. (For example, a 45-year-old woman will have an age score of 9 points and if she smokes needs to add an extra 11 points.)
At the end of the assessment total all the figures on the right to get your Total Risk Score. Then refer to table 6.

Risk Factor	Risk Points											Risk Score
Age (years)	35–39	40–44	45–49	50–54	55–59	60–64	65–69	70–74				
Age score	0	5	9	14	18	23	27	32				
Extra for smoker	13	12	11	10	10	9	9	8				

Systolic blood pressure (mmHg)	110–119	120–129	130–139	140–149	150–159	160–169	170–179	180–189	190–199	200–209	≥200
	0	1	2	3	4	5	6	8	9	10	11

Total Cholesterol (mmol/l)	≤5	5.0–5.9	6.0–6.9	7.0–7.9	8.0–8.9	≥9
	0	0	1	1	2	2

Height (m)	<1.45	1.45–1.54	1.55–1.64	1.65–1.74	≥1.75
	6	4	3	2	0

Creatinine (µmol/l)	<50	50–59	60–69	70–79	80–89	90–99	100–109	≥110	Don't know
	0	1	1	2	2	3	3	4	2

Risk Factor		Risk Score
History of heart attack	No = 0	Yes = 8
History of stroke	No = 0	Yes = 8
Thickened heart muscle	No = 0	Yes = 3
Diabetes	No = 0	Yes = 9
Taking anti-hypertensive medication	Yes = subtract 2 points from score	
	Total Risk Score	

Adapted from Pocock, S. J., et al. (British Medical Journal, 2001; 323: 75–81)

Table 5: Cardiovascular risk assessment (men)

For each row, choose the 'Risk Points' figure which corresponds with your own details and write it in the right hand 'Risk Score' column. (For example, a 45-year-old man will have an age score of 7 points and if he smokes needs to add an extra 7 points.) Note that 12 points are always added to male scores (first row).
At the end of the assessment total all the figures on the right to get your Total Risk Score. Then refer to table 6.

Risk Factor	Risk Points												Risk Score
Being male													12
Age (years)	35–39	40–44	45–49	50–54	55–59	60–64	65–69	70–74					
Age score	0	4	7	11	14	18	22	25					
Extra for smoker	9	7	7	6	6	5	4	4					
Systolic blood pressure (mmHg)	110–119	120–129	130–139	140–149	150–159	160–169	170–179	180–189	190–199	200–209	≥200		
	0	1	2	3	4	5	6	8	9	10	11		
Total Cholesterol (mmol/l)	≤5		5.0–5.9		6.0–6.9		7.0–7.9	8.0–8.9		≥9			
	0		2		4		5	7		9			
Height (m)	<1.60		1.60–1.69		1.70–1.79		1.80–1.89		≥1.90				
	6		4		3		2		0				
Creatinine (μmol/l)	<50	50–59	60–69	70–79	80–89	90–99	100–109	≥110	Don't know				
	0	1	1	2	2	3	3	4	2				
History of heart attack	No = 0						Yes = 8						
History of stroke	No = 0						Yes = 8						
Thickened heart muscle	No = 0						Yes = 3						
Diabetes	No = 0						Yes = 9						
Taking anti-hypertensive medication	Yes = subtract 2 points from score												
Total Risk Score													

Adapted from Pocock, S. J., et al. (British Medical Journal, 2001; 323: 75–81)

If you have not had your blood cholesterol checked in the past five years then it should be done – ask for your doctor to arrange it for you. At the same time it is easy for your kidneys to be checked with a creatinine level (it can be done on the same sample of blood) so ensure it is to be done too. If you have had a cholesterol check done in the past five years then that figure will be good enough, unless you have been taking treatment to lower it, in which case your most recent reading is the one you want.

Your doctor might have a cholesterol level recorded in your notes but possibly not a creatinine level. In that case you can use the average creatinine figure for your age to make the calculation – the details of what to do are within the tables. Note that table 4 is for women and table 5 is for men.

To use the calculator, work your way down the relevant table, noting your score for age, smoking history, blood pressure, cholesterol, height, creatinine, diabetes, past stroke or heart attack and heart enlargement. Add up your score and then look at table 6. The left hand column is your score, and against each figure there is percentage likelihood in the right hand column. This is an indication of your risk of suffering a *fatal* heart attack or stroke in the following five years. The figure below the table shows the same information graphically – find your score on the horizontal axis and go straight up to the curved line to find the risk figure on the vertical axis. Note that the curve increases steeply with higher scores.

One particular point that may have puzzled you is the lack of a question specifically on weight in this calculator. Increased body weight is associated with high blood pressure, raised cholesterol and the presence of diabetes and because each of these last three factors is included in the calculator, there is no obvious difference in the risk calculation when body weight is added. The message concerning weight is therefore hidden, but is nonetheless important – keeping body weight down is important in helping reduce the chance of developing conditions that increase the risk of developing cardio-vascular disease.

To use the tables effectively it is best to compare the effect of

Table 6: Risk score and probability of a fatal cardiovascular event in 5 years

Risk score	Percentage likelihood of dying from cardiovascular disease in 5 years
0	0.04
5	0.07
10	0.11
15	0.19
20	0.31
25	0.51
30	0.84
35	1.4
40	2.3
45	3.7
50	6.1
55	9.8
60	15.6
65	24.5
70	37.0

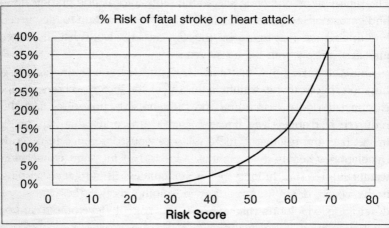

Adapted from Pocock, S. J., et al. (British Medical Journal, 2001; 323: 75–81)

changing modifiable risk factors *within each of the age bands*. Increasing age is the single biggest contributor to risk score for the obvious reason that as we get older we get nearer to the end of our lives. There is little point in a 60 year old comparing his or her risk with that of a 40 year old, as we can't make ourselves any younger – he should compare himself with another 60 year old. The following example illustrates the point.

Example
Imagine two 50-year-old men, both the same height at 1.75 metres, both with the same creatinine level of 80 µmol/l. Neither is diabetic. However, Man 1 smokes and has a raised blood pressure of 160 mmHg systolic, for which he does not receive treatment. His total cholesterol level is 6.2 mmol/l. Man 2 is a non-smoker and his systolic pressure is 126 mmHg and cholesterol level 4.8 mmol/l.

Counting up the risk points for Man 1 gives a total risk score of 43 and for Man 2 a total of 29. Referring to table 6, Man 1 has a five-year chance of a fatal heart attack or stroke of about 3 per cent – not a very high risk. Man 2 however has only a 0.8 per cent (approximately) chance of the same event. Putting it another way, Man 1 is over three times more likely to have a major cardiovascular event than Man 2 and all because of factors that are within his power to improve.

Stopping smoking reduces risk right away, but the fall is gradual and it is unclear how long it will take an ex-smoker's risk to drop to something near that of the person who has never smoked. It is however likely to be significantly lower by about two years after stopping. Blood pressure and cholesterol levels can be tackled and reduced over quite short time scales – a few months perhaps, with immediate improvement in cardiovascular risk. By taking anti-hypertensive treatment (–2 points), getting his blood pressure down to the 130–139 mmHg range (–3 points) and reducing his cholesterol to the 5.0–5.9 mmol/l range (–2 points), Man 1 will take his total score down to 36, which brings his chance of a stroke down to about 1.6 per cent – half of what it was. If he also stops smoking this will fall below 1 per cent within a few years.

Limitations of risk calculators

There are many limitations to using calculators such as this. For example this one does not take account of exercise level – not because it is unimportant (it certainly *is* important) but because it is hard to put a number against it that we could use in a formula. A person's family history of medical conditions such as high blood pressure, stroke, diabetes, etc is relevant, but with all the possible combinations that can result from the history of two parents with different ages, sexes and their own family histories it becomes too complex to add them to the calculation – so they are left out. This calculator attempts to calculate the risk of fatal heart attack or stroke – not minor ones that people can and do survive. Good diabetic care reduces complications but in these tables all diabetic people are grouped together, regardless of their diabetic state. Treatment of hypertension in people older than 74 is now known to be beneficial, but is not covered in the table – and so on.

In other words these tables have many limitations – but they are still useful guides to illustrate the impact of change. They can help to inform you about your state of health and what action might be worth taking to improve it, but they cannot tell you how fit you are, or cope with the particular details that make you unique. When you have the information from this risk calculation, please use it as a basis for discussion about your health with your doctor. You can't help being a man, for example, or make yourself any younger, but you can stop smoking, get some weight off, reduce your salt intake and take more exercise and each of these makes more of a difference than we can hope to calculate on paper. Risks tend to multiply but so do benefits – a little bit of improvement in each of the modifiable risk factors will benefit you significantly more than just one or two.

This calculator gives a five-year prediction for a fatal cardiovascular event. For a useful, free and easy to use calculator program for the ten-year risk of any heart attack or stroke (including minor events) see the British Hypertension Society's web site at http://www.hyp.ac.uk/bhs/managemt.html.

Key Points

- Several ways of calculating the risk of developing cardiovascular disease have been devised, but they should only be seen as a guide.
- Always compare risks within age groups, not between them.
- Because risks multiply each other it is better to achieve some improvement in several modifiable risk factors rather than concentrate on only one.

Chapter 8

The Treatment of High Blood Pressure

The fact that in so-called 'primitive' societies hypertension is virtually unknown reveals that in general high blood pressure is related to modern-day living. 'Essential' hypertension is a misnomer in this sense – there is probably nothing essential about the development of high blood pressure in human beings, yet it happens to at least 10 per cent of the adult western population. We are beginning to understand more of the puzzles that surround hypertension and know broadly how to treat it – but the success of that treatment depends in large part on the actions of the hypertensive person.

Certainly we now have a battery of powerful drugs for the condition, and a substantial proportion of people with hypertension need drug treatment no matter how hard they try to modify their lifestyle. But hypertension is not a problem for which drugs have the answer. No matter what the level of blood pressure is, or which drugs if any are being taken, there will always be positive benefits from improving diet, stopping smoking and taking exercise. For many people this is the only treatment they need.

'Lifestyle' treatment

SALT

We are a nation of salt addicts. The recommended total daily intake of salt for adults is 5 grams or less – a slightly heaped teaspoonful. Bearing in mind that this is to include all of the 'hidden' salt in processed and packaged foods, it leaves little room for the addition of salt at the table or in cooking. We can easily take two to four times as much salt as we need without trying because so much unnecessary salt comes to us in every variety of food.

Many of us add salt out of habit, and cutting it out is not easy at the start, but after a few weeks of restriction most people find it hard to believe how salty is the food that they had been used to eating. Leave the salt off the table, and cut the amount specified in recipes by half for a start. Fast foods such as hamburgers, preserved meats and fish, sausages, bacon, soy sauce, stock cubes, pickles, crisps and similar snacks are obvious sources but bread, tinned soups, microwave meals and a host of other foods may contain more salt than you think – a single slice of bread can contain 0.5 g of salt. It is worth noting how much sodium is present in what you buy and starting to look for lower salt brands. They are beginning to appear in greater numbers on supermarket shelves as the message begins to get through to the food industry that we want less salt. Sodium content may be marked as grams or as millimoles (mmol). The conversion is approximately 17 mmol per gram – so you are looking to get your daily intake to below 85 mmol of sodium. In Scotland for example the average 24-hour sodium intake (measured by collecting the amount passed in the urine) is 200–300 mmol – a marked excess over the body's needs.

Be careful, however, of using salt substitutes – these contain potassium chloride (table salt is sodium chloride). Potassium supplements are not suitable for people with impaired kidney function, or people receiving ACE inhibitor drugs or some types of 'water pills' (diuretics).

Both such types of drug are used in treating hypertension and are covered in more detail later in this chapter.

Salt reduction undoubtedly has a beneficial effect on the blood pressure of people with hypertension, and the impact is greater in adults over 45 and in people of African and Caribbean origin, who in general are more 'salt sensitive'. Evidence for the effect of salt on blood pressure came from the Intersalt study and the DASH-II (Dietary Approaches to Stop Hypertension) trial in the USA. In the DASH-II trial people were assigned to one of three diets whose sodium content was high (150 mmol/day), intermediate (100 mmol/day) or low (50 mmol/day). The difference in blood pressure observed between those on the highest and the lowest sodium-content diets was 12 mmHg, a response equal to that of potent anti-hypertensive drugs.

WEIGHT

Even modest weight loss makes a difference. Every pound (0.5 kg) lost drops blood pressure by about 1 mmHg and with a bit of help most people can comfortably lose 3 per cent to 9 per cent of their body weight. For someone overweight at 80 kg a loss of 5kg should be realistically achievable over a period of a few months, and could be expected to drop the blood pressure by 10 mmHg or more. In blood pressure terms, that is a substantial fall. It could make the difference between needing some drugs or none at all. Even if drugs are still required the dosage is likely to be less, and the likelihood of needing several drugs is reduced.

The healthiest way to lose weight is a sensible combination of diet and exercise. Exercise needs to be started at a low level – short walks for example – if you are out of condition, and increased slowly. If you have any doubts about your ability to start undertaking exercise you should ask your doctor for advice. Introduce dietary changes gradually too – you are trying to alter a habit in a way you can keep going with, perhaps forever. Crash diets don't work – they usually end up with you feeling weaker or giving up completely in desperation. This in turn can lead to a yo-yoing effect of weight loss/weight gain.

Eating 300 to 500 calories less per day may lead to losing between one and two pounds (0.5–1 kg) per week. This is a realistic rate of weight loss. It may seem slow, but if sustained would add up to more than 4 stones (26 kg) in a year. Having a glass of water instead of juice, eating less lunch than usual and having smaller portions of the food you enjoy are all ways to reduce calorie intake without having to necessarily alter your diet significantly. Avoid a second helping at dinner and snacks between meals, which may have become a habit. Cut down on beer and alcohol. All these things will influence your health in a positive way.

EXERCISE

Regular exercise does lower blood pressure but it is difficult to say by how much, because research studies done on exercise are usually combined with general lifestyle improvements rather than on exercise alone. Probably about a 5 mmHg drop in pressure is a fair estimate of what can be achieved. The level of exercise required to produce benefit is not excessive – a good walk or swim three times a week is enough to show results. Exercise has a definite benefit on overall cardiovascular risk. Those who exercise regularly and are fit (whether or not they have hypertension) have only a fraction of the risk (typically one half to one fifth) of similar people who take no exercise and are unfit.

POTASSIUM

Increasing the range and amount of fruit and vegetables in our diet has a range of benefits associated with the increased consumption of dietary fibre, vitamins and antioxidants (compounds which counteract the effect of 'free radicals' – highly reactive molecules that play a part in tissue damage and aging). Specifically as far as cardiovascular risk is concerned, fruit and vegetables are good dietary sources of potassium, and although high sodium intake is associated with higher risk of hypertension, high dietary potassium intake is associated with lower risk of hypertension.

Vegetables

Balance your vegetable intake between the orange/red and green varieties. As an easy rule the darker and brighter the colour of the vegetable the more vitamins, minerals and fibre it usually contains – compare lettuce with the deep dark green of spinach or the bright orange of carrots for example. The more starchy vegetables such as corn, butternut, pumpkin, peas, root vegetables and sweet potatoes should also be balanced with the less starchy vegetables such as courgettes, green beans, spinach, broccoli and cauliflower.

Aim for three or four portions of vegetables each day. One portion is:

- 1 cup of raw leafy vegetables
- ½ cup of other vegetables, cooked or raw
- ¾ of a cup of vegetable juice.

Try eating your vegetables raw as part of a sandwich filling or serve them with dips. You can make your own dip using yoghurt and finely chopped vegetables. Try juicing vegetables – they make a refreshing drink and, once prepared, it's a quick and easy way to increase your vegetable intake.

Microwave or lightly steam vegetables when cooking; this helps retain the nutrients, and makes preparation easier and less time consuming.

Fruit

To gain the maximum benefit from fruit, ensure that whenever possible it is fresh, and if the skins are edible, eat them too. Dried fruits and fruit juices can form part of your daily diet. However, they should be used in moderation, as fruit juices lose most of their natural fibre in the juicing process and dried fruits are high in carbohydrate (sugar).

Try to eat a minimum of three portions of fruit every day – more if you can. One portion of fruit is:

- 1 medium apple, orange, banana
- ½ cup chopped, cooked or canned fruit
- ¾ cup fresh fruit juice
- ¼ cup dried fruit.

Combine fruits like oranges and mangos in a liquidized fruit drink. Add chopped fresh fruit to your breakfast cereal or in yoghurt as a dessert.

FAT

High fat intake is associated with raised cholesterol in the blood and with increased cardiovascular risk. Fat is particularly high in calories, so reducing fat intake is a central part of weight-reducing diets. Whether high fat intake by itself raises blood pressure is uncertain but some evidence to suggest that it does came from the original DASH trial. In this trial three groups of people with high-normal blood pressure or mild hypertension were assigned to one of three diets – one was enriched with fresh fruits and vegetables, one was similarly enriched but also had low-fat dietary products and the third took a 'normal' diet. The lowest blood pressure readings were seen in the group who had increased fruit and vegetable intake combined with low-fat products.

Some fat is essential in our diet. Fats provide a source of concentrated energy and contain the essential fat-soluble vitamins A, D, E and K. The two main types of fat are 'saturated' and 'unsaturated'. Saturated fats are solid at room temperature and are the more undesirable from the health point of view. They are found mainly in lard, red meat, suet, dripping, eggs and full-fat dairy products. They are also found in hard margarines – which are often used for making cakes, biscuits and pastry. Avoiding these items will reduce your saturated fat intake considerably.

Unsaturated or 'good' fats are generally liquid at room temperature and come from vegetable sources but are also found in oily fish and in soft margarines labelled 'high in polyunsaturates'. These unsaturated fats contain essential fatty acids that cannot be manufactured by the body and need to be obtained from food. 'Omega-3' and 'omega-6' fatty acids are types found in oily fish and which appear to give additional protection against cardiovascular disease.

Some practical tips regarding dietary fat are:

- Choose lean meat or poultry, removing the excess fat before cooking.
- Try to reduce your intake of dairy products and eat more fat-free or soya based dairy products.
- Use semi-skimmed or soya milk in your tea, coffee and on your cereal.
- Avoid hard margarines, biscuits and pastries.
- Avoid frying and roasting foods – steam, grill, stir-fry and bake instead.
- Try to eat oily fish 2–3 times a week (herring, mackerel, mullet, salmon, trout, tuna, sardines, anchovies).

ALCOHOL
Consuming a small amount of alcohol daily (up to two standard units) appears to have a beneficial effect upon cardiovascular risk. There are many possible explanations for this, but among the most likely are that compounds within some alcoholic drinks, particularly red wine, mop up 'free radical' molecules that are capable of causing tissue damage. However, the effects rapidly turn from beneficial to harmful when higher levels of alcohol are consumed. Regular alcohol consumption raises blood pressure, particularly in individuals who are already hypertensive, but the effect wears off soon after the excessive drinking is curtailed. Binge drinking is associated with an increased risk of developing a stroke.

The usual recommended maximum consumption of alcohol per week is:

- 21 units for women
- 28 units of alcohol for men

but hypertensive people should limit their drinking to:

- 14 units per week for women
- 21 units per week for men.

(Source: British Hypertension Society guidelines)

A unit of alcohol is:

- 250ml (½ pint) of ordinary strength beer/lager
- 1 glass (125ml/4 fl oz) of wine
- 1 pub measure of sherry/vermouth (1.5 fl oz)
- 1 pub measure of spirits (1.5 fl oz).

SMOKING

Smoking has no effect upon blood pressure, but it has a marked effect upon cardiovascular risk and is the single biggest preventable cause of death in the UK. Stopping smoking is the top priority for any individual, and especially so for people with hypertension. Getting help to stop smoking is easier than it used to be. Nicotine replacement doubles a person's chance of quitting and medication such as amfebutamone (bupropion, Zyban) is also effective. Online support and information on stopping smoking is available free on NetDoctor at http://community.netdoktor.com/ccs/uk/smoking/index.jsp.

Drug treatment

Improvements in diet and exercise will always benefit health and to a greater or lesser degree will lower blood pressure but a proportion of people with hypertension will require drug therapy no matter how hard they try. Of these, less than half will be satisfactorily controlled on just one type of medicine, and a third will require three or more drugs.

Effective drugs for hypertension arrived in the 1950s and 1960s and although they had an immediate beneficial impact they also had many side effects which made them unsuitable for widespread use or for other than severe hypertension. Most of the drugs from that era are no longer used routinely. Modern therapy on the other hand is well tolerated and safe. With care it can be used in a very wide range of people of all ages.

DRUG CLASSES AND NAMES

We now have seven different 'classes' of drugs that can be used in treating hypertension:

- Diuretics
- Beta blockers
- Calcium channel blockers
- Angiotensin converting enzyme inhibitors
- Angiotensin receptor blockers
- Alpha blockers
- Other anti-hypertensive drugs.

Each class contains more than one drug but within each class the way in which the drugs work is essentially the same. All drugs have at least two names – the 'generic' name which is its officially recognised name and one or more 'proprietary' or 'brand' names given to the drug by different manufacturers.

When new drugs are formulated and marketed by a pharmaceutical company they are protected by patent for several years, during which time that company will be the only one producing the drug, so the drug will have only one proprietary name along with its single generic name. Once the patent on a drug runs out, other drug manufacturers can make and sell it, and they will often then give it their own proprietary names. Adding to the complexity of drug names is the commercial practice of combining more than one drug in one tablet. These combination drugs have some advantages, because it is easier to remember to swallow one pill rather than two for example, but as the dosage within the tablet is fixed they are less flexible in use. They also increase further the range of proprietary names. The names of drugs can therefore easily become very confusing. Generic names are used in this book when referring to drugs.

Unfortunately there is one more potential source of confusion concerning drug names, as generic names are currently changing to a European standard and this affects many of the names and spellings which have been in common use in the UK for decades (and are still the ones your doctor will be used to using!). Where there are differences the 'older' generic name will appear in this book in brackets after the 'new' one.

LIMITATIONS OF DRUG INFORMATION

In the rest of this chapter each class will be described. Full details of one representative drug from each class are listed in appendix B. There can be subtle differences between the drugs of any class so if you are taking one not described in this book it is important not to assume that the information will necessarily apply to you, other than in general terms.

The choice of a drug, its dose and the way it interacts with other drugs and medical conditions are matters for your doctor to discuss with you personally. The information provided here is intended to give you enough information for you to understand the broad principles of drug treatment for hypertension and to help you in your discussions with your doctor about your treatment. The information is not designed to provide a basis for a decision on any individual's medical care.

A full list of generic and proprietary names of all drugs currently in use in the UK, along with individual drug details, are in the medicines section of the NetDoctor web site at http://www.netdoctor.co.uk/medicines/index.shtml.

You may find it helpful to refer to chapter 2 for details of the biology of blood pressure control when considering how the different types of anti-hypertensive drug work.

THE MAIN CLASSES OF DRUGS USED IN HYPERTENSION

Diuretics

Diuretics are better known as 'water pills', referring to their ability to stimulate the kidneys to produce more urine. There are three types of diuretic in use for hypertension:

- Thiazide
- Loop
- Potassium-sparing.

Thiazide

The 'thiazides' are the commonest diuretics in use for hypertension. At the dosages used to lower blood pressure they in fact have only a mild effect on urine production but they do cause a gradual increase in loss of sodium, potassium and water from the kidneys, leading to a slow fall in blood pressure. They probably also cause some direct opening up of small arteries (arterioles) which adds to their blood pressure lowering ability. The two drugs commonly used in this class are bendroflumethiazide (bendrofluazide) and chlortalidone (chlorthalidone). Others include cyclopenthiazide, indapamide and xipamide.

Loop

Much less commonly used are the 'loop' diuretics (so called because they act upon a part of the kidney filtering mechanism called the Loop of Henlé). Loop diuretics are fast acting and powerful and are only used when there is a need to get rid of a lot of excess body water, such as occurs in heart failure for example. The three available are furosemide (frusemide), bumetanide and torasemide.

Potassium-sparing

The main two in this group are amiloride and triamterene. Whereas thiazide and loop diuretics tend to cause potassium loss as well as sodium loss from the kidneys, these two drugs do not. They are not used on their own to treat hypertension, but are combined with thiazides in some preparations to help reduce the potassium loss that can occur with thiazide diuretics. Now that we use lower doses of thiazides than we did some years ago potassium loss is less of a problem but for this reason amiloride and triamterene remain useful. However, their potassium-conserving power is a potential problem if they are given along with another class of anti-hypertensive drug – the ACE inhibitors – this can lead to dangerously high levels of potassium in the blood unless the dosages are monitored carefully.

Spironolactone

Spironolactone is also a potassium-sparing diuretic, but it has a unique action and is worth considering separately. It blocks the action of the hormone aldosterone, thus reversing the trend to retain sodium which aldosterone excess causes. It is not licensed for use in hypertension but has been shown recently to improve the survival of people suffering also from heart failure – which is commonly due to severe hypertension. Where excess aldosterone is being produced by over-activity or a tumour of the adrenal glands, spironolactone is the drug of choice. In fact adrenal surgery is now usually reserved only for those patients who are not adequately treated by spironolactone alone.

Diuretic usage

The thiazides, particularly bendroflumethiazide, are the most commonly used diuretics for blood pressure control. They are cheap and have been around a very long time, so we have a large amount of information on how they work and how best to use them. They are most useful in the elderly and in the black population, who seem more salt sensitive. The main problems with thiazides are: worsening of gout, diabetes and blood fat levels, lowering of blood potassium level and reversible impotence in men. Bendroflumethiazide is described in detail in appendix B.

Beta blockers

It was shown in the late nineteenth century that material extracted from adrenal glands would cause a rise in blood pressure if injected into an animal, and soon afterwards adrenaline was identified as the active substance. There are several adrenaline-like substances that are manufactured and used within the body as the chemical messengers of the sympathetic nervous system – noradrenaline is the other main one. Work done in the 1940s showed that these compounds acted upon two types of receptor molecules, named alpha and beta, which were present in different tissues and allowed adrenaline and noradrenaline to have different effects, depending on which receptors they met. Research then showed that there were actually subgroups of both types of receptor. Beta-1 receptors in the heart respond to adrenaline by increasing the heart rate and force of contraction, and beta-2 receptors in the airway tubes of the lung respond by opening the tubes wider.

Sir James Black won the Nobel prize in 1988 for his work at ICI in the 1950s and 60s which led to the invention of propranolol – the first beta-blocker drug. Beta blockers cause a fall in blood pressure, which is desirable, by acting on the heart's beta-1 receptors. However, their action on the beta-2 receptors of the lungs causes a narrowing of the airways of the lungs, which is of course undesirable. Much effort has gone into developing beta blockers specific to the heart which avoid problems in the lung but this has not been possible to achieve completely. People with asthma therefore need to avoid beta blockers, as they tend to make asthma symptoms worse. Beta blockers can, however, usually be used safely in other lung conditions, such as chronic bronchitis for example.

Beta blockers have been a mainstay of high blood pressure treatment and as they exert a 'braking' effect upon the heart they have also been very useful drugs in the treatment of angina – the condition in which chest pain develops on effort because of narrowing of the heart's own arteries. Use of beta blockers improves the outlook for people who have had a heart attack and in some people with heart failure. Although there are 16 different beta blockers currently available this includes some older ones no longer in regular use for hypertension. Those most commonly in present use are: atenolol, bisoprolol, celiprolol, labetalol, metoprolol and nebivolol. Atenolol is described in appendix B.

Side effects caused by beta blockers generally include: tiredness, slow pulse, cold hands and feet, worsening of wheeze, sleep disturbance and digestive system upset

Calcium channel blockers

The 'calcium channels' are the molecule-sized gates within the membrane of muscle cells. These gates control the flow of calcium ions in and out of the cell – when open they allow calcium to flood in, which triggers the muscle cell to contract. Blocking the channels causes the muscles that line arterioles to relax, thus making them wider, which lowers the resistance to blood flow and hence lowers blood pressure. Calcium channels within the heart are slightly different to those lining the arterioles, which is reflected in the fact that calcium channel blocking drugs can differ quite widely in their particular pattern of action. Verapamil and diltiazem, for example, have more effect upon the heart, where they reduce the heart's pumping ability. Amlodipine is now the most commonly used calcium channel blocker and is described in appendix B.

Other calcium channel blockers in regular use include felodipine, nifedipine, nicardipine and nisoldipine. All of the preceding calcium channel blockers may also be used to relieve the symptoms of angina. Others presently licensed only for hypertension are isradipine, lacidipine and lercanidipine.

Angiotensin converting enzyme inhibitors

Angiotensin converting enzyme (ACE) is present in lung tissue and converts circulating angiotensin I, which has no effect upon blood vessels, into angiotensin II, which has a powerful constricting effect and hence elevates blood pressure. ACE inhibitors block the production of angiotensin II and lower blood pressure very effectively. They have also proved very useful in the treatment of heart failure and in slowing the deterioration of kidney, eye and nerve function that can occur in hypertensive people who also have diabetes.

ACE inhibitors are well-tolerated drugs that can be given to a wide range of people. The most common side effect is a dry cough that can be troublesome enough to make the drug intolerable. It is caused by the action of ACE inhibitors on another enzyme within the lung. Very rarely a severe allergic reaction develops to ACE inhibitors.

In people who have unsuspected narrowing of the arteries to the kidneys as the cause of their hypertension (renal artery stenosis), ACE inhibitors can cause kidney function to get worse quickly. This can be avoided by checking kidney function with a simple blood test before starting an ACE inhibitor for the first time and then again one or two weeks later.

In the majority of people with hypertension an ACE inhibitor can be easily started and monitored by the general practitioner. Initial problems are more likely if the person is elderly or is already on high doses of diuretics, perhaps because of heart failure in which case smaller starting doses will usually get round the problem. Potassium-sparing diuretics can be used alongside ACE inhibitors, but caution is needed and more frequent blood checks on the potassium level have to be done.

Captopril was the first ACE inhibitor in regular use but requires to be given more than once daily and has been superseded by longer-acting drugs. These are: cilazapril, enalapril, fosinopril, imidapril, lisinopril, moexipril, perindopril, quinapril, ramipril and trandolapril. Lisinopril is the most commonly used ACE inhibitor and is described in detail in appendix B. All modern ACE inhibitors (i.e. other than captopril) can be given once daily and there is no difference between them in their potential to control high blood pressure.

A large trial of ramipril in people at high risk of developing cardio-vascular problems (HOPE – Heart Outcomes Prevention Evaluation study) reduced such events by 22 per cent and reduced the number of deaths from cardiovascular disease by 16 per cent. Although about half of the people in the trial had hypertension the amounts of blood pressure reduction were small, indicating the general effectiveness of

ACE inhibitors across the board in treating the effects of cardiovascular disease.

Angiotensin II receptor blockers

These drugs block the effect of circulating angiotensin II rather than reduce its production but in effect they reduce blood pressure in the same way as ACE inhibitors. Their main advantage is their remarkably low tendency to cause side effects. As they work outside the lung they do not cause cough, which can be a major advantage for some people. As yet they have not been shown to be superior to ACE inhibitors in treating hypertension but large studies investigating their role are under way.

The main precautions that need to be taken with ACE inhibitors should also be applied to the angiotensin II receptor blockers. The available drugs in this class are: candesartan, eprosartan, irbesartan, losartan, telmisartan and valsartan – which is described in appendix B. They can all be given once daily.

Alpha blockers

Blocking the alpha receptors of the sympathetic nervous system also causes widening of arterioles and a fall in blood pressure. Alpha blockers have been around for some time but were not particularly popular because they needed to be given frequently (two or three times daily) and could sometimes cause marked falls in blood pressure on standing (postural hypotension). Prazosin was the first alpha blocker in regular use and is described in appendix B.

Alpha blockers can slightly improve blood cholesterol levels and as new, longer-acting alpha blockers such as doxazosin and terazosin can be given once a day there has been a renewal of interest in using these drugs in hypertension. They are usually used as add-on treatment when blood pressure is difficult to control and not as the first choice or sole treatment.

Alpha blockers cause relaxation of the muscle which holds the bladder closed and which surrounds the prostate gland – a walnut-sized gland at the base of the bladder in men, through which urine passes on exit from the bladder. In all men it tends to get larger with age, and if it swells enough then it can make it harder for a man to pass urine.

Alpha blockers can therefore cause undesirable but reversible incontinence (bladder leakage) in women whereas in men with an enlarged prostate gland it can be a benefit, because the prostate's muscular coating relaxes a bit, allowing urine to pass through the prostate more easily. Because of the risk of a marked fall in pressure when first starting alpha blocker drugs the initial dose is kept small and people are advised to lie down until the first dose has had its effect. This problem usually disappears after the first few days of treatment.

OTHER ANTI-HYPERTENSIVE DRUGS
In this category are drugs used uncommonly in the UK or only in special circumstances. Brief details are given.

Vasodilators
These act directly on blood vessels to widen them:

- Hydralazine: effective by mouth and still a useful drug when combined with some others used for heart failure.
- Minoxidil: used in severe hypertension resistant to other drugs. Its side effect of hair growth makes it unsuitable for use in women but is exploited in the scalp treatment Regaine® which can temporarily improve male baldness. In this lotion form it does not lower blood pressure.
- Diazoxide and sodium nitroprusside: rarely used drugs which can be used by injection for severe hypertension.

Centrally acting drugs
'Centrally acting' means that these drugs work on the chemical messenger links between nerves within the sympathetic nervous system. The result is a drop in activity of the sympathetic nervous system and a fall in blood pressure.

- Methyldopa: still used for severe hypertension in pregnancy because it is probably safe for the foetus.
- Clonidine: in smaller doses than those used for hypertension clonidine can help flushings associated with the menopause. It needs to be stopped slowly to avoid 'rebound' increase in blood pressure.
- Moxonidine: a more recently invented drug with a possible role where other drug therapy has failed, but it can cause drowsiness.

All centrally acting anti-hypertensives should be avoided in depression.

CHOOSING THE RIGHT DRUG

The object of drug therapy is to achieve target blood pressure levels using the minimum number of drugs and to minimise side effects at the same time. Side effects from medicines tend to occur in proportion to the amount of each drug being used, so it is often better to use two drugs at low dose than to stick with one and have to increase its dosage to a level at which side effects start to occur. In any case some anti-hypertensives, such as thiazide diuretics and beta blockers, work best at low dosage and their effects are not increased by greater dosage.

It is often necessary to combine anti-hypertensive drugs. Three quarters of people needing drug treatment for high blood pressure will need to combine two or three to get the desired effect. Tailoring medication to fit the individual requires skill and it can take some time – months easily – to find the right balance. No matter which drug is used, lifestyle improvements will always help reduce blood pressure and are an essential part of hypertension treatment.

Figure 13 is a flow diagram showing some of the possible options that can guide the initial choice of drug, and it is not as complex as it may appear at first. Starting at the 'hypertension' box and following through the choices for someone who does not have extra factors such as heart failure, diabetes, angina or a previous heart attack leads to the thiazide diuretics – the preferred initial choice in 'straightforward' essential hypertension.

Figure 13: Flow chart for initial drug choice in hypertension

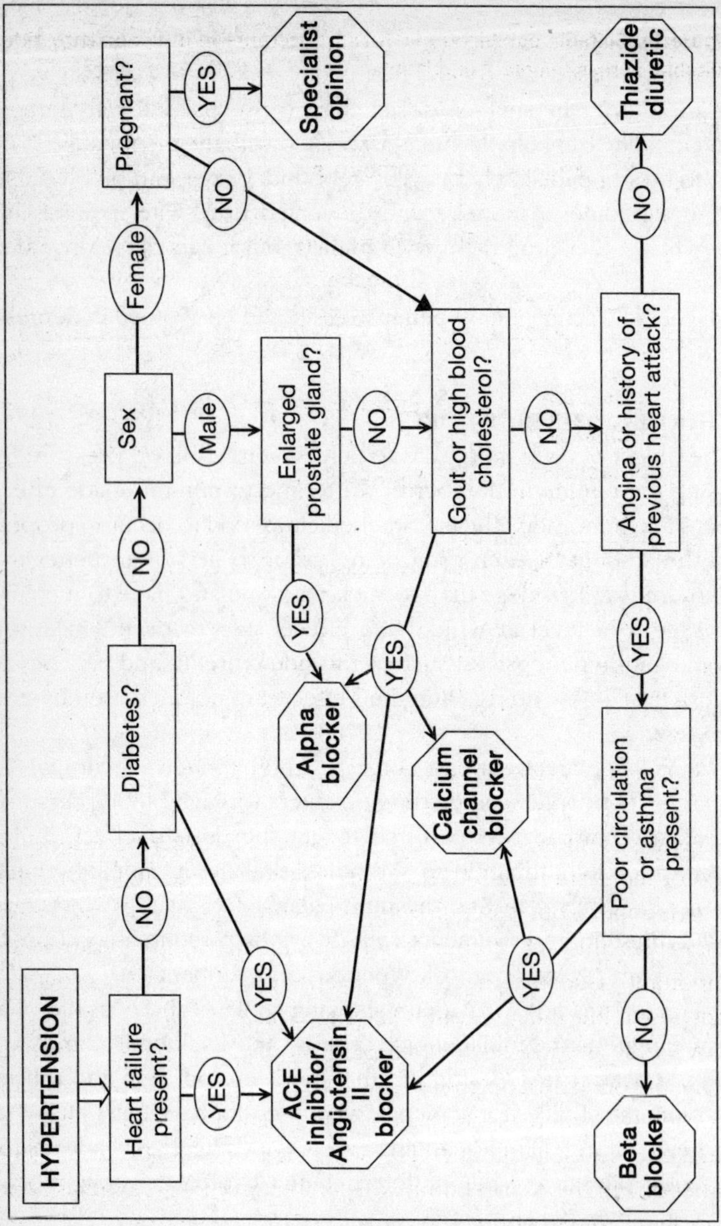

Figure 14: Suitable combinations of anti-hypertensive drugs (side to side = suitable; across middle = unsuitable)

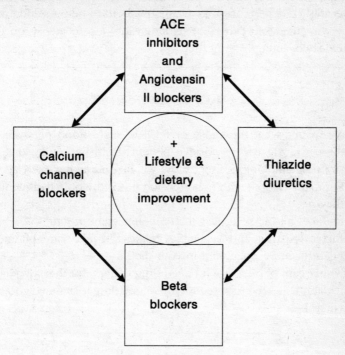

Figure 14 shows preferred combinations of drug to be used when two or more are required. Each class will combine well with either of its neighbours, but less well with a class on the other side of the circle. Charts like this are of course only a guide and cannot address every important issue that needs to be considered in prescribing for an individual, but they are a fair starting point.

A handy alternative way of looking at this is the 'ABCD' method. In general, younger people respond better to an ACE inhibitor (A) or beta blocker (B) whereas older people do better with calcium channel blockers (C) or a diuretic (D). When it comes to combining drugs either one of the A or B group will combine well with either one of the C or D group. So you could have (A+C), (A+D), (B+C) or (B+D).

Despite the best efforts of the general practitioner and patient alike some people have high blood pressure that is difficult to control. Then the specialist in hypertension is invaluable, both to help exclude rare or otherwise treatable causes of hypertension and to advise on the complexities of multiple drug therapy.

Key Points

- No matter what the cause or level of high blood pressure, there will always be positive benefits from improving diet, stopping smoking, losing excess weight and taking exercise.
- For many people with hypertension this is the only treatment they need.
- Reduce salt intake to less than 5 grams daily *in total*.
- Increasing fruit and vegetable intake will take care of the need for more potassium in your diet.
- 75 per cent of people who need drug therapy for their hypertension will need to take more than one drug to achieve good control.

Chapter 9

Blood Pressure in Special Groups

Elderly people

The observed rise in blood pressure with age (figure 3, see p 8) used to be taken as a sign that high blood pressure was something to be accepted in older people and that it did not need to be taken so seriously as hypertension in the young. This is now known to be incorrect. The age-related rise in pressure is not seen in tribal populations who consume less salt than westerners and the SHEP study (Systolic Hypertension in the Elderly Program) showed clearly that the treatment of high blood pressure in the elderly gave substantial protection against strokes. Later results from the SHEP group also showed that heart failure is prevented by treating hypertension. The development of dementia is also probably slowed by good control of blood pressure.

The implications of achieving the blood pressure levels we now believe to be necessary in people over 60 (maximum 160 mmHg systolic and 90 mmHg diastolic) are quite staggering. As many as half of the population over 60 may be hypertensive by this definition, and therefore need treatment. The evidence in favour of treating high blood pressure in the elderly extends at least as far as people up to the age of 80, and may well extend to older people too – research into this is well under way. Increasing numbers of people now live to their eighties and beyond and it is clear that the detection and treatment of hypertension is a major public health problem.

PRACTICAL BLOOD PRESSURE PROBLEMS WITH ELDERLY PEOPLE

Unfortunately the evidence is that within the National Health Service we still have a very long way to go to detect and treat hypertension adequately – in all age groups, but particularly in the elderly. Many doctors still hold very cautious views on the definition of and need to treat hypertension in people over 60. Such caution need not, however, be fuelled by anxiety that older people cannot tolerate high blood pressure treatment adequately – they do so very well.

Two other reasons why hypertension in the elderly has taken something of a back seat in importance relate to a) practical difficulties with diagnosis and b) the condition of systolic hypertension. Both of these will now be explained.

As we get older the elasticity of our blood vessels falls. They become a bit more rigid, and this makes it easier for them to conduct sound waves. This in turn affects the Korotkov sounds, upon which the measurement of blood pressure depends. Normally the disappearance of the sound of the pulse is taken as the diastolic pressure reading – the low point in the blood pressure cycle before the next heart beat. However when the blood vessel walls are more rigid, the sound may persist, even if the pressure is dropped all the way to zero. This makes it difficult or impossible to accurately judge the correct diastolic pressure. Another fairly common difficulty in assessing the pressure accurately arises if there is a pulse abnormality called 'atrial fibrillation'.

In this condition, which is quite common in older people, the atria beat out of step with the ventricles. This leads to some beats when the ventricles are not fully charged with blood, so the strength of each pulse varies and this makes accurate readings difficult.

The second difficulty is a condition, almost exclusively found in elderly people, in which the systolic pressure can be high despite a normal diastolic blood pressure reading. This is called 'systolic hypertension', and it used to be considered to be another consequence of old age and artery hardening, and not very important. We now know this to be incorrect, and that systolic hypertension is an equally important 'risk factor' for the development of a stroke or heart attack, and it needs to be treated just as vigorously as any other pattern of hypertension. Systolic hypertension is however more difficult to treat – it can be harder to get the systolic pressure down without causing side effects from treatment such as dizziness on standing up. This has influenced medical practice towards caution in the past but we now have to accept that systolic hypertension matters, and needs to be dealt with in its own right.

Choosing the appropriate drug in the elderly follows the same principles outlined in chapter 9, and in figures 13 and 14 (see pp 102–103). The thiazide diuretics are the drugs of choice, and calcium channel blockers next if thiazides are unsuitable or inadequate, along with attention to diet and exercise within reasonable limits.

Diabetes

There are two main types of diabetes – Type 1 is that found in younger people (under 35 approximately) and is due to insufficient or absent production of the hormone insulin by the pancreas gland inside the abdomen. Insulin is necessary to control the body's use of glucose – the main energy source for our tissues.

In both types of diabetes the typical symptoms include thirst, frequent passage of urine, tiredness, tendency to thrush infection and weight loss. Type 1 diabetes always causes enough symptoms to get noticed and needs to be treated with insulin injections. Type 2 diabetes is much more common, and occurs in people of middle age or older. They tend to be overweight and essentially do not produce enough insulin for their needs. As many as half of the people who have Type 2 diabetes are unaware of it – their symptoms may be so mild they do not seek medical advice for them until years later. Type 2 diabetes can be treated by diet alone, or by diet plus tablets to lower the blood sugar.

In both types of diabetes better control of the blood sugar lowers the chance of long term problems especially to the eyes, kidneys, heart, brain and nerves. The ACE inhibitors seem particularly helpful in hypertension associated with diabetes (mostly Type 1, less so for Type 2), slowing the rate at which long-term kidney damage might occur.

In Type 1 diabetes, provided the condition is well controlled and there are no kidney complications, high blood pressure occurs with about the same frequency as in non-diabetic people. In Type 2 diabetes, however, as many as 70 per cent or more of those with the condition will also be hypertensive. In all people with both diabetes and hypertension good blood pressure control reduces the risk of long-term tissue damage. In diabetes all cardiovascular risk factors are magnified in effect, so particular efforts need to be made to reduce excess weight, lower blood cholesterol if it is high and to take more exercise – a high proportion of people with Type 2 diabetes are both overweight and sedentary.

Diabetes is a very important condition, which is getting commoner and is associated with significant health problems if poorly treated. The reverse side of the coin is that with care and attention to detail, and rigorous blood pressure control, complications from diabetes should be rare. British Hypertension Society guidelines are that all diabetic people should aim for blood pressures consistently less than 140/80 mmHg. Some other expert groups advocate an even tighter target of 130/80.

Pregnant women

As women in their reproductive years who take the contraceptive pill will have their blood pressure checked regularly there is more chance that a young woman with hypertension will be detected than a young man, but sometimes a rise in blood pressure in a woman will be detected for the first time during the course of her pregnancy. A pregnant woman is as likely as any other woman her age to develop essential hypertension, unrelated to the pregnancy itself, and we assume that women who show a rise in pressure during the first half of pregnancy (up to 20 weeks) have essential rather than pregnancy-related hypertension. That should be investigated along the same lines as outlined in chapter 6. In pregnancy blood pressure over 140/90 mmHg is considered high and many specialists would act on lower levels than this, as blood pressure normally falls in pregnancy, increasing the significance of raised readings.

PRE-ECLAMPSIA

Pregnancy is however associated with a unique blood pressure problem, called pre-eclampsia, that can develop any time but is much commoner in the second half of pregnancy (20 weeks onwards) and up to a week after delivery. It occurs in about 5 per cent of first pregnancies, but any pregnant mother can develop it. In pre-eclampsia the mother's blood pressure rises, she develops puffiness of the face, hands and feet, and her kidneys become 'leaky' – losing excess amounts of protein. The degree of pre-eclampsia can vary between mild, requiring careful observation and perhaps deliberately inducing labour a bit early but no other treatment, to severe, with the need for vigorous blood pressure treatment or emergency delivery if the baby appears at significant risk. Fortunately pre-eclampsia rarely becomes severe enough to result in eclampsia – an epileptic fit brought on by the high blood pressure and other complex changes that occur in the mother's body in this condition.

Although we do not fully understand why pre-eclampsia occurs many details are known. The placenta is the attachment point of the baby to the mother's womb and is rich in blood vessels that come very close to, but remain separate from, the mother's circulation. Oxygen from the mother passes to the baby through the placenta, and waste carbon dioxide from the baby goes into the mother's bloodstream. In pre-eclampsia there is distortion and narrowing of these tiny blood vessels, which reduces the capacity of the placenta to nourish the baby. In many ways the behaviour of the mother's immune system during pregnancy is quite remarkable. Normally any complex living being, such as a person, will detect and react against invaders such as bacteria, or protein from another person that does not match their own. A child grows of course from within the mother's body but in many ways is completely different to the mother, yet she tolerates the presence of this 'foreign body' for nine months. One of the theories explaining pre-eclampsia is that this mother-baby tolerance mechanism breaks down slightly and the blood pressure rise is a sign of it.

Regular blood pressure checks are therefore a routine part of ante-natal care, along with weight checks and urine tests for protein – these are easily done with 'dipsticks'. A minor technical problem often arises in pregnancy in the measurement of the blood pressure as the diastolic pressure can be difficult to read (as in elderly people, but for a different reason). Therefore the muffling of sounds heard with the stethoscope (Phase 4 Korotkov sound) is used in place of the disappearance of sound (Phase 5). This also means that automatic blood pressure machines may not give reliable blood pressure checks and when in doubt a mercury or aneroid sphygmomanometer should be used to check the pressure.

Pre-eclampsia is said to be present if any one or more of these things happen during the pregnancy:

- Rise in systolic pressure of 30 mmHg or more
- Rise in diastolic pressure of 15 mmHg or more
- Diastolic pressure greater than 90 mmHg on two occasions or 110 mmHg on one occasion
- Excess protein in the urine.

The symptoms of pre-eclampsia include swollen feet and hands, head-aches, flashing lights or blurred vision and tummy pains but they do not always occur together. Also, not every headache in pregnancy means pre-eclampsia is occurring. Should any woman experience these symptoms she should always check with her midwife or doctor that all is well.

TREATMENT

The treatment of high blood pressure in pregnancy is a specialised subject and requires close co-operation between the midwife, the GP and the obstetric specialist. Many specialists will treat a mother whose blood pressure is at or greater than 140/90 mmHg, and specialist advice should certainly be sought in any pregnant woman with blood pressure of this level, at any time in the pregnancy.

The choice of drugs available in pregnancy is severely limited by safety considerations for the unborn baby, and no drug is known to be completely safe. Drugs which must be avoided include ACE inhibitors, angiotensin II blockers and most beta blockers, although some are used – labetalol and atenolol in particular. Thiazide diuretics tend to be avoided because of concerns that they will reduce the flow of blood to the placenta, but there is no definite evidence that they are unsafe in pregnancy. Experience over many years has shown that methyldopa is usually safe, as well as the alpha blockers. The calcium channel blockers are usually best avoided but one of them (nifedipine) has been used in severe pregnancy hypertension.

Unfortunately dietary salt restriction is ineffective in lowering blood pressure in pregnancy and is not recommended. Taking some rest is a good idea, as is ensuring a reasonable amount of exercise, but taking an excess of either does not lower blood pressure. Most hypertension problems in pregnancy are nonetheless managed easily – it is very unusual for significant problems to arise in either mother or baby with modern obstetric care. The important points are to attend for regular antenatal checks, to be sensible about diet, exercise and rest and to stop smoking.

Ethnic groups

People from either an Afro-Caribbean or Indian origin show an increased tendency to develop hypertension and its complications. In a study of ethnic groups in south London up to half of Afro-Caribbean people over 40 had high blood pressure. In Indian populations diabetes is very common, of the 'Type 2' variety – the type that is largely controllable by diet.

Why these variations occur is not fully understood. It seems that blacks are more 'salt sensitive' than other ethnic groups, which also means that salt restriction is more effective in them as a measure to lower blood pressure. Traditional Indian diets are high in hard fats – the 'saturated' type, which we know are associated with hardening of the arteries in the body. A high proportion of people from Indian backgrounds who live in the UK are overweight and take inadequate amounts of exercise, both of which increase the likelihood of heart disease and diabetes occurring.

As far as anyone with hypertension is concerned – no matter what their ethnic origin – the message concerning high blood pressure remains the same. Lifestyle factors are very important and are the mainstay of treatment. On top of that there are minor points that need to be borne in mind regarding the use of drugs – for example ACE inhibitors on their own are not so effective in black people – but provided these are remembered there is no reason why the results of hypertension treatment should differ between people of different race. Hypertension is a treatable disorder in all human beings who develop it.

Low blood pressure (hypotension)

Although this book is concerned with the special problems associated with high blood pressure, low blood pressure – hypotension – also exists and has its own associated causes and problems. There are however marked differences in the way hypotension is diagnosed and treated in Britain and the USA compared to mainland Europe – particularly France and Germany.

Among British and American doctors, the term hypotension is restricted to the situation in which a person's blood pressure is low enough to cause symptoms such as dizziness on standing too quickly. Such a problem – called postural hypotension – is recognised as a side effect of treatment of hypertension in the elderly for example.

Among doctors in mainland Europe, however, the diagnosis of

hypotension is made with much greater frequency, and hypotension is blamed for a range of symptoms including fatigue, dizziness, headache and low mood. In a survey comparing German and British general practitioners' surgeries, 17 per cent of German patients were reported 'hypotensive' either by themselves or by their GP. The proportion of women was twice that of men, and it was commoner in the young. A quarter of these patients were on treatment to raise their blood pressure. In contrast, the diagnosis of hypotension is virtually never made in UK general practice to explain fatigue, and almost no British doctor would prescribe for it – even if there were safe and effective medicines available to do the job – which there are not.

There is some evidence to suggest an association between tiredness and low blood pressure but it is unclear how important the observation is, and very uncertain that attempts to raise blood pressure would be in any way beneficial. As far as UK practice is concerned, therefore, hypotension is a diagnosis made in specific physical situations and is not generally accepted as the cause of otherwise unexplained fatigue.

Other situations

INSURANCE

For many people the first time they will have a full medical examination, or perhaps even a blood pressure check, will be at a medical examination for an insurance company. These are common when taking out life insurance cover, for example in association with a large loan such as a mortgage. Often your own general practitioner can do them, and it can certainly help to make you feel relaxed if the person doing the examination is known to you, but they do tend to be stressful occasions. In such circumstances an elevation of blood pressure is likely to reflect anxiety to a large extent.

Unless your blood pressure is very high at the examination and there are other medical reasons to suspect that it has been elevated for a while, then any high readings should be repeated several times. This is good practice in any case, and most insurance companies accept the need for repeat readings, but there can be practical difficulties in getting them done. It may be difficult for you to get time off, for example, or the doctor you see could be someone from another practice, in a different town, or from a private health company and repeat appointments may be difficult to arrange. Ask the doctor or nurse checking your pressure at such a medical what the readings are. If they are high then insist on repeat readings. Of course you may need to accept that you do have high blood pressure, once it has been fully assessed and properly investigated, but if so you will probably need to pay more for your insurance, so it is worth ensuring that the readings reflect your true blood pressure. It is worth checking the particular rules that an individual insurance company applies (if they will discuss them), as some will not increase the premium if the blood pressure is under good control on treatment.

DRIVING

The UK regulations for ordinary car drivers require notification to the Driver and Vehicle Licensing Authority (DVLA) only if the treatment of high blood pressure gives rise to symptoms which would affect safe driving. Other than that, the DVLA need not be notified if you have hypertension. Holders of commercial driving licenses need to notify the DVLA if their systolic pressure is consistently 180 mmHg or above, or diastolic 100 mmHg or above. Once the pressure is controlled, and provided the treatment does not influence safe driving, then the license will be returned.

FLYING

There are no particular factors you need to worry about when flying if you have hypertension and are taking effective treatment. Flying does make some people especially anxious, and temporarily therefore causes blood pressure to rise, so if you have very high blood pressure which is proving difficult to control, and particularly if you do get anxious on flying, you should discuss your situation with your own doctor beforehand.

HOLIDAYS

In very hot climates it is natural to sweat a lot and sweat contains salt, so some increase in salt and fluid intake is required to compensate. If you are on a restricted salt diet to control your blood pressure then some relaxation of the diet might be advisable while in hot countries. You would be likely to know that your blood pressure was falling too low if you began to feel dizzy on standing. A minor adjustment of drug dosage might be required – but this needs your doctor's advice.

It is easy to forget to pack medicines when going on holiday. Anti-hypertensive drugs need to be continued long term, but little harm will usually result from missing a few doses if your hypertension is mild. It is not a good idea to go a week or longer without medication, so it's important to take adequate supplies of medicine to cover the whole holiday, and perhaps some extra to cope with delays. Although the medicines commonly used for hypertension are widely available within Europe, North America, Australia and New Zealand (the names may differ but the active ingredient is the same) some of the more recent drugs may be hard to find in other countries, so don't rely on buying medicines abroad.

Key Points

- Hypertension can and should be treated in people up to the age of 80 years at least.
- Good blood pressure control in diabetes reduces the long-term complications that diabetes can cause.
- Hypertension in pregnancy poses special problems but can usually be well controlled, thus avoiding complications for the mother and baby.
- Black populations tend to be more at risk from hypertension, and more responsive to reducing salt in the diet.

Chapter 10

The Challenge of Hypertension

High blood pressure is the commonest treatable medical condition in the developed world – around 15-20 per cent of the middle-aged population and about 50 per cent of those over 60 have mild to moderately raised blood pressure and 5 per cent of the adult population have significantly raised blood pressure. We are, however, not doing well in treating it.

The situation was put succinctly thirty years ago as 'The Rule of Halves':

- Half of all people with hypertension have been diagnosed
- Half of those known about have been treated
- Half of those treated are treated inadequately.

Some improvement has certainly occurred – for example The National Health and Nutrition Examination Surveys (NHANES), which are large population surveys undertaken in the USA, showed the proportion of people with blood pressures over 140/90 fell from 36 per cent in 1974 to 20 per cent in 1991. Even allowing for differences in the measuring techniques used, this seems to indicate that we are getting better at recognising and treating hypertension. However, the NHANES III information also showed that whereas 60 per cent of white women on hypertension treatment had their blood pressure controlled at the target of 140/90 mmHg, only 47 per cent of black men had theirs controlled.

There is no room for complacency in Britain either. For example, a survey of nearly 8000 men from 24 towns throughout Britain showed a threefold variation in the number of men diagnosed with hypertension, with a trend towards higher rates in Northern England and Scotland. Only one quarter of men with high blood pressure could recall having been diagnosed as hypertensive by a doctor, and only one third of these were on regular anti-hypertensive treatment.

At the present time the resources and organisation within the National Health Service are inadequate to ensure that all healthy adults are chased up to have a blood pressure check every five years (as recommended by the British Hypertension Society) or annually for those who show high normal values, nor is a faultless service provided to those people diagnosed with hypertension. We are not alone – a recent survey within Europe showed that less than 30 per cent of hypertensive people were well controlled.

Hypertension is very much a community problem, and one that ought to be dealt with well by primary care – general practitioners and their associated colleagues. The reality that we are doing badly at detecting and treating it does not reflect the level of education and expertise of British doctors and nurses (which is very high), nor a lack of awareness on their part of hypertension's importance (this is widely acknowledged), nor the cost of the treatment (many of the drugs effective in hypertension are cheap). The problems lie at a more basic level within the structure of the National Health Service – it was built not as the means by which the public's health would be actively encouraged to improve, but as a system of access to medical care for the sick.

When the NHS as we now know it was born in 1948, Bevan ensured it was possible for general practice to flourish on the basis of local doctors with lists of patients in defined geographic areas. This led the way for continuity of care, which is one of the undoubted strengths of the British system of medicine. The ordinary citizen could obtain the services of a doctor without paying a fee, and it was indeed an out-standingly successful innovation.

At that time the population's health was seen as a battle largely won. Mortality from common illnesses was a fraction of what it had been a hundred years earlier due to massive improvements in living conditions, water and food supplies, and sanitation. The advent of antibiotics in the 1940s seemed to herald an age in which medical advances would wipe out all illness. The focus, however, was very much on the treatment of disease within hospitals. By contrast general practice was the unglamorous face of medicine, usually looked down upon by specialists and shunned by the best medical graduates who were attracted to brighter lights and higher rewards.

Those attitudes have changed and primary care is now seen in its proper light as the only setting in which the biggest challenge – improving the health of the population – can occur. Unfortunately we still have an organisational structure within primary care that has hardly changed in half a century. In particular, Community Medicine (as Public Health is now called) has remained a small medical specialty with few consultants and with no staff teams of their own to carry out major screening programmes or health education. Community Medicine acts mainly as an advisor to primary care which has the job of carrying out public health policy, but which is unequipped for the task. It is an unsatisfactory situation for everyone – for the person with undiagnosed or under-treated hypertension who may suffer avoidable ill-health, for the health care teams who take no pleasure in dealing with the consequences rather than the causes of illness and for society as a whole, as the burden of ill health is one we all need to carry.

Programmes to improve public awareness of hypertension (and diabetes, and the other public health issues that affect us) need much more attention than they have received in the past. The NHS has not achieved these population-sized goals, but it was never designed to do so. A major shift is needed in attitude and commitment if real improvements are to be made in the health of the people of this country. The biggest changes we need to make are not in waiting lists or access to high-technology medicine, but in the basics of how we live.

One of the most important ways in which improvement can be encouraged is for the public to become better informed in health matters and join the discussion. Historically this has not happened and many decisions of fundamental importance to our health have been, and continue to be, made without adequate public dialogue. One of the aims of this book is to help you engage in those debates. You can also do your bit for the public good by passing the message on to others who might not yet have heard it – check your blood pressure.

Key Points

- Hypertension is a major public health problem that is dealt with poorly within the UK.
- The majority of people who have hypertension are either not yet diagnosed or are inadequately treated at present.
- More resources are certainly needed to tackle hypertension but public attitude is also important, as much can be done to reduce the chance of hypertension occurring by simple lifestyle measures that everyone can follow.

Appendix A

References

Risks of high blood pressure

1 Framingham Heart Study; http://www.nhlbi.nih.gov/about/framingham/
2 'MRC trial of treatment of mild hypertension: principal results' (British Medical Journal, 1985; 291: 97–104).
3 Pocock, S. J., et al., 'A score for predicting risk of death from cardiovascular diseases in adults with raised blood pressure, based on individual patient data from randomised controlled trials' (British Medical Journal, 2001; 323: 75–81); http://bmj.com/cgi/content/full/323/7304/75
4 MacMahon, S., et al., 'Blood pressure, stroke and coronary heart disease, Part 1' (Lancet, 1990; 335: 765–74).
5 Kannell, W. B., Hypertension: physiopathology and treatment. (McGraw Hill, New York, 1977).

ELDERLY PEOPLE

1 Bulpitt, C. J., et al., 'The Hypertension in the Very Elderly Trial (HYVET)' (Journal of Human Hypertension, 1994; Aug 8(8): 631–2).

2 SHEP Co-operative Research Group, 'Prevention of stroke by anti-hypertensive drug treatment in older persons with isolated systolic hypertension: Final results of the Systolic Hypertension in the Elderly (SHEP) program' (Journal of the American Medical Association, 1991; 265: 3255–64).

3 Kostis, J. B., et al., 'Prevention of heart failure by anti-hypertensive drug treatment in older persons with isolated systolic hypertension in Europe' (Journal of the American Medical Association, 1997; 278: 212–6).

4 Forette, F., et al., 'Prevention of dementia in randomised placebo-controlled systolic hypertension in Europe (SystEur) trial' (Lancet, 1998; 352: 1347–57).

5 Lever, A. F., and Ramsay, L. E., 'Treatment of hypertension in the elderly' (Journal of Hypertension, 1995; 13: 571–9).

6 Kostis, J. B., et al., 'Does withdrawal of antihypertensive medication increase the risk of cardiovascular events? Trial of Nonpharmacologic Interventions in the Elderly (TONE) Cooperative Research Group' (American Journal of Cardiology, 1998; Dec 15 82(12): 1501–8).

SALT

1 Intersalt Co-operative research group (British Medical Journal, 1988; 297: 319–28).

2 He, J., et al., 'Relation of electrolytes to blood pressure in men: The Yi people study' (Hypertension, 1991; Mar 17(3): 378–85).

3 The Trials of Hypertension Prevention Collaborative Research Group, 'Effects of weight loss and sodium reduction intervention on blood pressure and hypertension incidence in overweight people with high-normal blood pressure: The Trials of Hypertension Prevention, phase II' (Archives of Internal Medicine, 1997; Mar 24 157(6): 657–67).

Populations and ethnic groups

1 NHANES III study; http://www.cdc.gov/nchs/nhanes.htm
2 Weinberger, M. H., 'Salt sensitivity of blood pressure in humans' (Hypertension, 1996; 27: 481–490); http://hyper.ahajournals.org/cgi/content/full/27/3/481
3 Cappuccio, F. P., et al., 'Prevalence, detection and management of cardiovascular risk factors in different ethnic groups in south London' (Heart, 1997; 78: 555-63); http://www.sghms.ac.uk/depts/gp/WHSS.htm

Guidelines for blood pressure management

1 Ramsay, L. E., et al., 'Guidelines for management of hypertension: Report of the third working party of the British Hypertension Society' (Journal of Human Hypertension, 1999; 13: 569–92); http://www.hyp.ac.uk/bhs/1000917.pdf
2 'Recommendations for routine blood pressure measurement by indirect cuff sphygmomanometry' (American Journal of Hypertension, 1992; 5: 207–9).

Blood pressure measuring devices

1 Ashworth, M., et al., 'Sphygmomanometer calibration: A survey of one inner-city primary care group' (Journal of Human Hypertension, 2001; Apr 15(4): 259–62).
2 O'Brien, E., et al., 'Blood pressure measuring devices: Recommendations of the European Society of Hypertension' (British Medical Journal, 2001; 322: 531–6); http://bmj.com/cgi/content/full/322/7285/531

Standards of medical care

1 Mashru, M., and Lant, A., 'Interpractice audit of diagnosis and management of hypertension in primary care: Educational

intervention and review of medical records'. (British Medical Journal, 1997, 300: 981–3); http://bmj.com/cgi/content/full/314/7085/942

2   Dickerson, J. E. C., and Brown, M. J., 'Influence of age on general practitioners' definition and treatment of hypertension' (British Medical Journal, 1995; 310: 574); http://bmj.com/cgi/content/full/310/6979/574

3   Wilber, J. A., and Barrow, J. G., 'Hypertension – a community problem' (American Journal of Medicine, 1972; 52: 653–63).

4   Ritchie, L. D., and Currie, A. M., 'Blood pressure recording by general practitioners in North East Scotland' (British Medical Journal, 1983; 286: 107–9).

5   Heller, R. F., and Rose, G. A., 'Current management of hypertension in general practice' (British Medical Journal, 1977; 1: 1442–4).

6   Shaper, A. G., et al., 'Blood pressure and hypertension in middle-aged British men' (Journal of Hypertension, 1988; May 6(5): 367–74).

7   Wilhelmsen, L., and Strasser, T., 'WHO-WHL hypertension management audit project' (Journal of Human Hypertension, 1993; 7: 257–63).

Diet

1   Sacks, F. M., et al., (New England Journal of Medicine, 2001; 344: 3–10 (Dash 2)); http://www.psychiatry.wustl.edu/Resources/Literature List/2001/February/Sacks.pdf

2   Appel, L. J., et al., 'A clinical trial of the effects of dietary patterns on blood pressure' (New England Journal of Medicine, 1997; 336: 1117–24); http://content.nejm.org/cgi/content/abstract/336/16/1117

Exercise

1   Halbert, J. A., et al., 'The effectiveness of exercise training in lowering blood pressure: A meta-analysis of randomised controlled trials of 4 weeks or longer' (Journal of Human Hypertension, 1997; 11: 641–9).

2 Engstrom G., et al., 'Hypertensive men who exercise regularly have lower rate of cardiovascular mortality' (Journal of Hypertension, 1999; 17: 737–42).

Alcohol

1 Kaplan, N. M., 'Alcohol and Hypertension' (Lancet, 1995; 345: 1588–9).
2 Gill, J. S., et al., 'Stroke and alcohol consumption' (New England Journal of Medicine, 1986; 315: 1041–6).

Drug therapy

1 Pitt, B., et al., 'The effects of spironolactone on morbidity and mortality in patients with severe heart failure' (New England Journal of Medicine, 1999; 341: 709–17).
2 Yusuf, S., et al., 'Effects of an angiotensin converting enzyme inhibitor, ramipril, on cardiovascular events in high-risk patients' (New England Journal of Medicine, 2000; 342: 145–53 and 748). (HOPE Study)
3 Brown, M. J., et al., 'Optimisation of antihypertensive treatment by crossover rotation of four major classes' (Lancet, 1999; 353: 2008–13). (ABCD method of drug selection)

Low blood pressure

1 Donner-Banzhoff, N., et al., 'Hypotension – does it make sense in family practice?' (Family Practice, 1994; 11: 368–74).
2 Wessely, S., et al., 'Symptoms of low blood pressure: A population study' (British Medical Journal, 1990; 301: 362–5).
3 Pilgrim, J. A., et al., 'Low blood pressure, low mood?' (British Medical Journal, 1992; 304: 75–8).

Appendix B

Anti-hypertensive drugs – class examples

Only brief details of each drug are given here. Full details are included in the manufacturer's data sheets and can also be viewed within the medicines section of the NetDoctor website http://www.netdoctor.co.uk/medicines/

The information is accurate at the time of writing but new information on medicines appears regularly. A health professional should always be consulted concerning the prescription and use of medicines.

Medicines and their possible side effects can affect individual people in different ways. The following lists some of the side effects that are known to be associated with these medicines. Side effects other than those listed may exist.

Thiazide diuretic – bendroflumethiazide

HOW DOES IT WORK?

Bendroflumethiazide is one of a group of drugs called thiazide diuretics. These stimulate the kidneys to increase the removal of salts such as potassium and sodium from the blood. This in turn causes water to be drawn out of the blood and into the kidneys, where it is then excreted in the urine. Removing water from the blood decreases the volume of fluid circulating through the blood vessels, which helps to lower high blood pressure.

MAIN SIDE EFFECTS

- Thirst
- Muscle cramps
- Digestive upset such as diarrhoea, constipation, nausea, vomiting or abdominal pain
- High blood uric acid level, which can cause gout
- Dizziness on standing due to a temporary fall in blood pressure
- Disturbances in the levels of salts in the blood
- Increased production of urine
- Blood disorders such as a low white cell count (rare)
- Rash
- Reversible inability of a man to have an erection (impotence).

OTHER MEDICINES CONTAINING THE SAME ACTIVE INGREDIENTS

Neo-Naclex

Beta blocker – atenolol

HOW DOES IT WORK?

Atenolol belongs to a group of medicines called beta blockers. These block the action of two chemicals called noradrenaline and adrenaline that occur naturally in the body.

Their action on the heart causes it to beat more slowly and with less force. The heart therefore uses less energy and the pain of angina is prevented. Abnormal heart rhythms are also prevented or reduced. Due to the reduced heart pumping action the pressure at which blood is pumped out of the heart to the rest of the body is reduced.

MAIN SIDE EFFECTS
- Headache
- Slow pulse
- Dry mouth
- Changes in mood
- Fatigue
- Digestive upset such as diarrhoea, constipation, nausea, vomiting or abdominal pain
- Dizziness
- Wheeze or breathlessness due to narrowing of the airways
- Dizziness on standing due to a temporary fall in blood pressure
- Spasm of the blood vessels of fingers and toes and cold extremities
- Cramping pain in the leg (calf) muscles on exertion
- Rash.

OTHER MEDICINES CONTAINING THE SAME ACTIVE INGREDIENTS
Tenormin preparations

Calcium channel blocker – amlodipine

HOW DOES IT WORK?
Amlodipine belongs to a group of medicines called calcium channel blockers. These dilate the blood vessels in the body and are used to treat high blood pressure and angina.

Amlodipine slows the movement of calcium through muscle cells in the walls of blood vessels. Calcium is required for these muscle cells to contract, thus amlodipine causes the muscle cells to relax. This causes the blood vessels to dilate.

Blood pressure depends on the force with which the heart pumps the blood, and on the diameter of blood vessels and the volume of blood in circulation. Blood pressure increases if the blood vessels are narrow or if the volume is high. Dilating the blood vessels in the extremities therefore decreases blood pressure.

The coronary arteries in the heart are also dilated by amlodipine, and this allows more blood, and therefore oxygen, to be delivered to the heart at any time. Overall the heart is required to use less effort to pump blood around the body, and is also given a greater oxygen supply. This prevents the pain of angina, which would normally be brought on because of a lack of oxygen supply to the heart.

MAIN SIDE EFFECTS
- Headache
- Rash
- Increased blood flow to the skin (flushing)
- Reversible inability of a man to have an erection (impotence)
- Nausea
- Fatigue
- Dizziness
- Fluid retention causing, for example, puffy ankles
- Weakness or loss of strength
- Enlargement of the gums.

OTHER MEDICINES CONTAINING THE SAME ACTIVE INGREDIENTS
Istin

Angiotensin converting enzyme inhibitor – lisinopril

HOW DOES IT WORK?

Lisinopril belongs to a group of medicines called ACE inhibitors, which block the action of an enzyme in the body called angiotensin converting enzyme (ACE). ACE is involved in the production of another chemical, angiotensin II. Thus lisinopril reduces the amount of angiotensin II in the blood.

Angiotensin II has two actions. Firstly it acts on blood vessels to make them narrow and secondly it acts on the kidney to produce less urine. As lisinopril blocks the production of angiotensin II, these actions are reversed. Therefore the kidneys produce more urine, which results in less fluid in the blood vessels. The blood vessels also widen. The overall effect of this is a drop in blood pressure and a decrease in the workload of the heart.

MAIN SIDE EFFECTS

- Dry cough
- Rash
- Fast pulse
- Dry mouth
- Reversible inability of a man to have an erection (impotence)
- Confusion
- Digestive disturbances such as diarrhoea, constipation, nausea, vomiting or abdominal pain
- Severe swelling of lips, eyes or tongue (angioedema)
- Dizziness
- Alteration in taste
- Heart attack (myocardial infarction)
- Profound drop in blood pressure (hypotension)
- Stroke (cerebrovascular accident)
- Disorders of the blood, kidney or liver
- Decreased kidney function.

Angiotensin II receptor blocker – valsartan

HOW DOES IT WORK?

Valsartan belongs to a group of medicines which block angiotensin II receptors in the body and prevent a naturally produced compound called angiotensin from working.

Angiotensin II has two actions. Firstly, it acts on blood vessels to make them narrow and secondly it acts on the kidney to produce less urine.

As valsartan stops angiotensin II from working, these actions are reversed. Therefore the kidneys produce more urine, which results in less fluid in the blood vessels. The blood vessels also widen. The overall effect of this is a drop in blood pressure.

MAIN SIDE EFFECTS

- Fatigue
- High blood potassium level
- Severe swelling of lips, eyes or tongue (angioedema)
- Dizziness
- Nosebleeds (epistaxis)
- Decrease in the number of a type of white blood cell (neutrophil) in the blood (neutropenia).

OTHER MEDICINES CONTAINING THE SAME ACTIVE INGREDIENTS

Diovan

Alpha-blocker – prazosin

HOW DOES IT WORK?

Prazosin belongs to a class of medicines called alpha blockers. It works by blocking the effects upon certain tissues and nerves of two naturally occurring compounds – adrenaline and noradrenaline. Blocking these receptors within the walls of blood vessels causes the muscles to relax, making the blood vessels wider and lowering blood pressure. Widening of the blood vessels also decreases the effort required by the heart to pump blood around the body, as there is less resistance. This can help treat heart failure, where the pumping action of the heart has become less effective.

Alpha receptors are also present on the muscle covering the prostate gland. This gland is found only in men and lies at the base of the bladder. Urine from the bladder has to flow through the prostate gland initially. The prostate gland often enlarges with advancing age (benign prostatic hyperplasia) and can cause urinary symptoms such as poor flow of urine. By blocking the alpha receptors, prazosin causes the muscle in the prostate to relax. This allows urine to flow more freely past the prostate and relieves the urinary symptoms.

MAIN SIDE EFFECTS
- Headache
- Depression
- Dizziness on standing due to a temporary fall in blood pressure
- Drowsiness
- Digestive disturbance such as diarrhoea, constipation, nausea, vomiting or abdominal pain
- Weakness
- Awareness of the heartbeat (palpitations)
- Fluid retention causing, for example, puffy ankles
- Incontinence
- Erectile problems in men – either reversible inability of a man to have an erection or a persistent painful erection of the penis (rare).

OTHER MEDICINES CONTAINING THE SAME ACTIVE INGREDIENTS
Hypovase

Appendix C

Useful addresses

British Heart Foundation

Major UK charity supporting all aspects of research into cardiovascular disease and providing a wide range of information for the public.

England and Wales
14 Fitzhardinge Street
London W1H 6DH
Tel: 020 7935 0185
Fax: 020 7486 5820

Scotland and Northern Ireland
45a Moray Place
Edinburgh EH3 6BQ

Tel: 0131 225 1067
Fax: 0131 225 3258
Website: www.bhf.org.uk
Email: internet@bhf.org.uk

The High Blood Pressure Foundation

Scottish charity existing to improve the basic understanding, assessment, treatment and public awareness of high blood pressure, and, in so doing, help promote the welfare of people with high blood pressure.

Department of Medical Sciences
Western General Hospital
Edinburgh EH4 2XU
Tel: 0131-332-9211
Fax: 0131-537-1012
Website: www.hbpf.org.uk
Email: hbpf@hbpf.org.uk

The Blood Pressure Association

A forum for individuals whose lives are affected by blood pressure, drawing attention to the importance of high blood pressure and trying to ensure better detection, management and treatment. Registered charity.

60 Cranmer Terrace
London SW17 0QS
Tel: 020 8772 4994
Fax : 020 8772 4999
Website: www.bpassoc.org.uk

British Hypertension Society Information Service

The internet information service of the main medical society for hypertension experts in the UK. Also contains information for the public.

Website: www.hyp.ac.uk/bhsinfo/

PubMed

The National Library of Medicine's on-line database of medical journal articles. Free to search over the internet.

Website: www4.ncbi.nlm.nih.gov/PubMed/

Omron Healthcare (UK) Ltd

Manufacturers of blood pressure measuring devices.

19–20 The Business Park,
Henfield BN5 9SL
Tel: 01273 495 033
Fax: 01273 495 123